# All of a Piece

# All of a Piece

## A Life with Multiple Sclerosis

BARBARA D. WEBSTER

THE JOHNS HOPKINS UNIVERSITY PRESS
BALTIMORE AND LONDON

The Johns Hopkins University Press
701 West 40th Street   Baltimore, Maryland 21211
The Johns Hopkins Press Ltd., London
"paperback edition 1998"
"0-8018-6162-4(pbk)"
*The paper used in this publication meets the minimum requirements of American
National Standard for Information Sciences—Permanence of Paper for Printed
Library Materials, ANSI Z39.48-1984.*

LIBRARY OF CONGRESS CATALOGING-IN-PUBLICATION DATA
Webster, Barbara D.
All of a piece : a life with multiple sclerosis /
Barbara D. Webster.
p.    cm.
Bibliography: p.

1. Webster, Barbara D.—Health.   2. Multiple sclerosis—
Patients—United States—Biography.   I. Title.
RC377.W43   1989
362.1'96834'0092—dc19
[B]                          88-29343
CIP

*For N and for P*

# Contents

# Foreword

I recently had the opportunity to address an audience of several hundred people, most of whom had multiple sclerosis, about new research findings in the disease. About half were visibly limited by their MS: they used canes or crutches, walkers, wheelchairs, or electric scooters. The master of ceremonies—a courtly gentlemen deeply interested in MS, but without the disease himself announced the opening of the program with the request that all present stand for the presentation of the colors, the flags of the United States and of the state, by a local scout troop. The impact was palpable: you could feel in the air the embarrassment, frustration, and anger of those in the audience who could not respond to this simple patriotic request because of the limitations their MS had imposed upon them.

For me, this event summarized much of what it must mean to be chronically ill in America today. In this age of modern medicine, we too often tend to think of serious chronic disease in terms of medical and scientific "breakthroughs," but rarely in terms of the human dimension and the relationship of illness to the cultural setting in which an affected person must exist.

In the above drama, a well-intentioned individual acted without thinking about the limitations of his audience; he probably is still not aware of his gaffe. Yet no one in the audience could reasonably call him down; it would have been "unseemly" to do so. Rather, they simply had to accept the reality of the situation—a reality about which they have learned, in most cases, after years of dealing with MS.

Acceptance is a key theme in this highly personal essay by Ms. Webster. In her terms, acceptance means acknowledgement of the conflicts that our culture and society create for chronically ill people and the realization that such conflicts will continue. Importantly, acceptance here does *not* imply that the conflict—or its impact—will be eliminated, nor does it preclude anger at the circumstances that generated the conflict. This is a highly humane kind of acceptance, and one that doesn't box a person into an unreasonable "never-never-land" existence.

Barbara Webster has multiple sclerosis—a fairly benign case of it by her own estimation. Her struggle with MS is fairly typical: a young woman with poorly defined symptoms bounces from doctor to doctor, with no good evaluation of what is happening and no diagnosis. Years go by, with friends and family becoming increasingly suspicious of her "sickness"; psychiatry is recommended. Finally, the diagnosis comes: multiple sclerosis. This pattern is one which many people with MS will recognize and with which they will identify.

For Ms. Webster, the diagnosis some five years ago was a "watershed" and has opened up a floodgate of highly personal reflections about herself, her disease, and her relationship to her loved ones and to society. While much of the book is clearly a self-exploration, there is no question that many people with MS and other chronic, disabling diseases will share the same feelings and reactions: she has written what many must feel but are unable to express.

There are key concepts and words repeated throughout the book: hope, denial, acceptance, uncertainty, vulnerability, dependence, adjustment. These are the issues that Ms. Webster confronts—issues she might never have had to face without the added life-burden of MS. While there are no answers here, the book is thought-provoking and probing, and forces the reader to consider critically the lot of a large segment of our population today. Chronically ill people will benefit from Ms. Webster's sharing; "outsiders" will learn about an aspect of life they may never have to face and will profit by that new knowledge.

STEPHEN C. REINGOLD, PH.D.
*Assistant Vice-President for Research and Director of Grants Management, National Multiple Sclerosis Society, New York City*

# Acknowledgments

I would like to thank Kevin Avruch, who first suggested that there might be a book here and whose interest and guidance were invaluable. Without him, I would not have begun this project.

Pat Nicolette lived through much of this experience with me, and he knows well what he has been for me.

Peter Black has been a constant source of support and encouragement. He patiently and carefully read each succeeding draft, of which there were many. His thoughts are interwoven with mine. Any remaining suggestion that culture is a moving force, however, is mine alone.

I would like to thank my hosts in Israel and Egypt, Bill and Sandra Brew. Without them, I never would have seen the Middle East.

Sar Levitan put food on my table (as he might say), introduced me to Jack Goellner, and is a wonderful friend and inspiration.

Jack Goellner has been the kind of editor I always imagined. His encouragement and belief that there really was something worth working on here kept me going. Whenever I felt like giving it up, one of his wonderful letters would arrive.

# All of a Piece

# Wrestling with a Phantom

*There's the whole question, which interested me . . .*
*of the things one doesn't say; what effect does that have?*
*. . . And then there's the question of things, happening,*
*normally, all the time.*
VIRGINIA WOOLF

A few years after discovering that I have multiple sclerosis, I visited Egypt with a friend. There I had an experience that remains a metaphor of much of my experience with MS. We found ourselves one day at the airport in Luxor on our way to Cairo.

The word "airport" is something of a misnomer; I was reminded of an old and little-used branch railroad station. There was one room and one small ticket window. Jammed into this very hot and airless little room were hundreds of people, few of whom seemed to know what was going on. My friend and I eventually checked in for our flight to Cairo (although that, too, conveys a false impression of order and efficiency) and, by comparing our boarding passes with others, got at the end of what seemed to be the proper line.

Nothing happened. It soon became obvious that no one was going anywhere any time soon and that the line was essentially irrelevant. We spotted some empty seats and started working our way toward them through the crowd. Suddenly I was pushed hard, lost my balance, and fell. We realized that we were in the midst of a group of elderly American tourists, all with name tags, who were loudly objecting to our presence in their area and actually pushing us away. "Who do they think they are? They don't belong with us. They are pushing into our line. Why does she have a cane—there's nothing wrong with her." They were quite amazingly nasty and, in the center of this scene of very Egyptian absolute and seemingly uncontrolled chaos,

1

had created their own bit of America. The contrast was compelling. They wanted to know exactly when the flight was leaving and the answer, of course, was always the same—*Insh'allah* ("God willing" or "when God wills"), which infuriated them. They would not yield an inch of their fiercely guarded territory.

Faced with a total inability to control what was going on, they were going to extreme lengths to foster their sense of being in control. They seemed to think that continually fighting for a place in this largely illusory line would get them to Cairo faster. My friend and I, on the other hand, having accepted that we had no control in this situation, were beginning to revel in that feeling; the mood is very catching and, after all, did it matter if we ever got to Cairo? We were more concerned with waiting, being there in some comfort while they, faced with chaos, fought ever harder to maintain the illusion of doing something by pushing and pulling in line. And that, of course, was why there were empty seats for us.

My experience with MS is first and foremost a personal story. It is rooted in my history and my personality. Much of what I have found most difficult—and the metaphor for that is being pushed around by those rude Americans in Luxor—is a personal issue and something, no matter its source or explanation, for me to come to terms with. But it became increasingly clear to me that taken out of the context of the society I live in and the cultural framework through which meaning is created, there was limited adaptive power to be found in my personal story. The meaning of disability and chronic illness and many of the consequences of those states are socially determined. It took me a while to realize that. Initially I thought that coming to terms with having a chronic disease was an individual task, one to be undertaken in isolation. But chronic disease is not just defined by society, it is experienced through the mediating structures of society and culture.

The scene at the airport in Luxor began to seem a paradigm for me of that juxtaposition—that relationship. Me set alongside, and in, a society that gives its own sets of meaning to my experience. It was the very starkness of the contrast—that reconstruction of America set down in the midst of Egypt—that was so revealing and that allowed me to begin to see my own experience in a larger context. And it was that context, together with my own story, which ultimately provided some illumination and eased the process of coming to terms with having a chronic disease.

My experience with multiple sclerosis began long before I ever associated the name with myself. When I was twenty-three, in the late 1960s, I was hospitalized for a week-long battery of neurological tests. Over the previous six months, I had experienced a host of symptoms. I had recurring urinary tract infections, balance and vision problems, difficulty with walking and with my speech, and extreme fatigue. The speech problem was frustrating. It involved knowing exactly what I wanted to say and being unable to articulate it. There were also times when I was physically unable to form words. The most problematic symptom for me was that I was completely unable to walk in a straight line. I always veered right and routinely walked into walls. Negotiating the sidewalks of Manhattan was difficult, to say the least. I was forever having to stop and move back into the center of a sidewalk. At my office, where I was a litigation paraprofessional in a law firm with long narrow corridors, people joked about my bouncing off the walls as I walked (if it could be called that) from one place to another.

I saw a doctor, who spoke of overwork and resulting exhaustion and treated some of my symptoms. Essentially, however, he seemed to think that because there was no readily apparent reason for my complex of symptoms, there was nothing wrong with me. The only problem with that diagnosis from my point of view was that I did not get well; I became increasingly weak and my symptoms became more and more pronounced. It was very difficult for me to function on a day-to-day basis.

Eventually, and I think partly in order to protect himself—even in the late 1960s doctors were concerned about malpractice suits—my doctor said that one possible explanation for all these symptoms was a brain tumor and recommended a neurological workup to rule out that possibility. Because my family knew a well-regarded neurologist at a medical center near their home, it was decided that I would go there for these tests. I say "it was decided" purposely. By this time I was not functioning well at all and merely acquiesced in the decisions others made for me.

In the hospital I had what felt like every medical test known to man, from brain scans—the old-fashioned kind—to electro-encephalograms to elaborate vision tests. I was visited by heart specialists and virologists. The most frightening test and, after the fact, the most interesting, was a brain angiogram. Dye is injected through an artery in the neck, and pictures are taken as the dye flows through the brain. Because this was a teaching hospital and angiograms were rarely done on one so young, there was a large crowd squeezed into a small room, all, it seemed, looming over me as I lay there. There was difficulty in-serting the needle into my neck, and I went into shock. That increased the uneasiness I had begun to feel when I had been required to sign a special release form for the procedure. What was fascinating, and frightening, was the feeling as the dye flowed through my brain—one never feels one's brain, but sud-denly it was a palpable reality. Because dye was injected only into the left side of my brain, I could feel that and, at the same time, not feel the right side. It was both terrifying and exhila-rating. I also felt as though I must squeeze my eyes shut to keep this hot, surging liquid from escaping from my head. It was al-together an amazing experience.

At the end of all these tests I was told that there was a faint but unlikely possibility that I had had a virus which had since disappeared. The doctors' best judgment was that there was nothing organically wrong with me, and that I had some kind of unspecified nervous disorder. I was told to rest for a couple of months, and that because there was no medical reason for what had been happening to me, there must be an emotional reason. It was "all in my head." It was also pointed out to me that one good reason for my illness could be found in the circumstances of my life. At that time I was seriously involved with Nick, the man I was later to marry, and I was told that this relationship was making me sick, and that unless I ended it I would get sick again. At that time, Nick was still married to his first wife, and I was violating all sorts of social canons by my involvement with him. This was, after all, 1969. I had no intention of ending this relationship and I felt that, given the undercurrents of disapproval emanating from my family, my illness was being used as a way to exert pressure on me. There was some reason for this feeling; the messages I was receiving were confused—nervous disorder, emotional reasons (I was simply neurotic), my relationship with Nick.

On the day that I was discharged from the hospital there was a blizzard, and, because my family could not pick me up, old friends took me to their house to spend the night. They were very kind and acting, I am sure, from good intentions, talked incessantly about how wrong Nick was for me. Nick was also stranded because of the blizzard, but I was not allowed to see him. It may sound strange that I, at twenty-three, allowed myself to be not allowed to do something. But I remember the feeling of extreme powerlessness I had at that time and I was very unwell and had no strength. What strength I had I used to insist that I would not end this relationship.

The next day my father arrived to drive me home and talked about the changes I needed to make in my life. In the car, he commented that my jaw was set and that I was being very stubborn. A set jaw describes perfectly how I felt; I felt very alone, very misjudged, and determined to hold to my own sense of who I was and what was right for me. I knew that there was something definitely wrong with my body but there was no one at that stage, with the exception of Nick, who agreed with me. I felt as though I was alone in front of a wall of figures endowed with expertise and authority who were all saying that I was wrong. From my perspective, the central fact, the central reality in all of this, was that no one trusted me; my family and friends tended to trust others—the voices of medical authority and knowledge.

At this time, it was strongly suggested that psychiatric help was in order. After all, I was sick and if there was nothing wrong with my body there must be something wrong with my mind. My doctors very explicitly said: "We can find nothing wrong with you, therefore there is nothing wrong with you. If you do not get well, that means there is a psychological cause for your illness." I was also gravely warned that unless I "worked through my problems," I would get sick again.

I was very resistant to the idea of psychiatric help but eventually agreed to see someone. I went back to New York, where I lived, and started trying to find a psychiatrist. After being interviewed by a couple of psychiatrists who seemed unsympathetic and unhelpful, I simply refused to see one. Beyond the fact that I saw no reason to engage in that exercise, it seemed very clear to me that the explanation for walking into walls was not to be found in the far reaches of my childhood.

I did slowly recover my strength; my symptoms abated entirely with time and, after a couple of months, I began working again. This episode left me uneasy, however, and uncertain. I had to doubt my own instincts to some degree because I received almost no support from anyone. Could I really believe that I was right and everyone else wrong? I did say that but mainly to myself, and there were many moments when I doubted my perceptions.

I felt uncertain vis-à-vis those close to me because they seemed to accept the notion that it was all in my head. I felt that people saw me as unstable and perhaps neurotic. People did not trust me to know what was going on in my own body. They listened, instead, to the experts and the experts had dismissed me. I hesitated to mention or complain about any physical ailments because I doubted they would be seen as legitimate. I was very reluctant to see a doctor for the most simple thing because I was afraid I would be seen as a hypochondriac or as simply hysterical.

After I said no to psychiatric help, it seemed to me that I was viewed as both denying that I had an emotional problem and being unwilling to do the "hard work"—that phrase beloved of therapists—necessary to deal with my problems. I felt very strongly that, seen through the eyes of others, there was an element of choice in my weakness because I had rejected the recommended and available fix.

I did get well again, however, and except for the lingering

and profound effects on my relationships, the episode seemed closed. I seemed to tire more easily and had little stamina; otherwise all the symptoms disappeared. I resisted as best I could the effects on me of what other people thought. With the single exception of Nick, who seemed simply to accept that I lacked stamina and respected my obvious limits, most people treated me as though any weakness was illegitimate and, being a reflection of some emotional deficiency, to be ignored. It was not a valid reason for anything.

Four years later, when Nick and I were living together, I got sick again. "Aha, we were right all along." And because there was now a history of my being "sick" with no reason, the scenario was repeated, except that this time less effort was made to find a physical cause, and I was more quickly referred to a psychiatrist. I was told that I was clinically depressed and that my symptoms were a result of that depression.

The symptoms this time included recurrent urinary tract infections and a borderline hyperactive thyroid. My legs were extremely weak, which made walking at times almost impossible. I had bouts of incredible fatigue in which it seemed I would never be able to move again. I soon learned that a thyroid problem is one of those ailments that is not seen as discrete but as tending to involve psychological problems. What luck. In any event, treatment of the thyroid did not cause my symptoms to abate. I also, almost overnight it seemed, became extraordinarily sensitive to heat. I could no longer tolerate heat and humidity at all; my weakness and shakiness increased dramatically. It seemed clear to me that there was something radically wrong with my body, but again I received little support for that notion. I don't recall whether at the time I connected this episode with the earlier one except in terms of its emotional consequences. New doctors, on hearing my medical history (or lack of *medical* history), seemed quicker to assert that there was nothing wrong with me. Those close to me, again with the exception of Nick, concurred.

And I had been warned four years earlier that unless I accepted that there was a psychological reason for my problems, I would get sick again. I had gotten sick again. It was becoming very hard for me to continue to believe in my own interpretation of what was happening to me. Again, no one trusted me, and that lack of trust and the sense I had of being railroaded led to a deep and resounding sense of betrayal by some of those who were close to me.

Primarily out of a sense of deep exhaustion and because I felt very alone, I agreed to see a psychiatrist. I would have agreed to almost anything. My level of despair and my sense of helplessness were so high by this time that I might well have been clinically depressed. I tend to think, however, that I was just extremely frustrated. I was certainly unhappy about being so sick, knowing that, whatever the cause, there was clearly something wrong with my body, and receiving no support from anyone.

I soon found myself in the classical box of Freudian psychology: until you admit that we are right, you are wrong. I asked what seemed to me the obvious question, "What if I never do agree that you are right, what then?" "Then," I was told, "that will prove we are right." I would not be emotionally healthy until I admitted there was a psychological cause for my physical problems. My refusal to acknowledge that was a confirmation as far as they were concerned, another pathological sign.

The fact that I would not admit that I was clinically depressed (and I think in retrospect it is clear that I was not) confirmed them in their belief that I was. The fact that I clearly was not very happy about any of this was also seen as confirmatory. I found the whole situation very depressing indeed, and it was difficult to maintain a sense of integrity in the face of all this disapproval and certainty.

An event occurred during this time that was so extreme and so absurd that it actually increased my sense of integrity and affirmed my belief in my own perceptions about what was happening to me. It also increased my distrust of psychiatrists and my belief that they can do a great deal of damage on occasion. I had made an appointment with a psychiatrist. When making it I had told him that perhaps it would be better to postpone it because my car was being worked on that morning and I was not sure it would be finished in time. He said no, if I had to postpone at the last minute that would be OK. It became appar-

ent that morning that the car would not be ready in time and so
I called to cancel the appointment. The doctor said, "Don't cancel it, just call when you are ready." So I called later on and he
said, "OK, I'll see you when you get here."

When I got to his office, he began to scream at me (and there
is no exaggeration here) for being late. I said, "Wait a minute. I
am not late; we changed the appointment." And he went on to
talk about how I (someone he had seen once before for an hour
when I had been punctual) was chronically late and how that
indicated my hostile and manipulative nature and, moreover,
that I expected the whole world to bow to my whims. I found
myself on the defensive (a big mistake) and said, truthfully, that
I was almost never late for anything. He then accused me of
being a pathological liar. He went on to say that I was clearly
suicidal and no doubt had often attempted suicide in an attempt
to gain attention. By this time, I was in a state of shock—this
man knew nothing about me and was apparently drawing all
these conclusions from my "lateness." I was rarely late; I had
never considered suicide. He continued to yell at me and said
that undoubtedly I would successfully kill myself. At that point,
I recovered my wits and said I was leaving. As I walked out,
a gust of wind blew through the open window and the door
slammed shut behind me. As I walked down the hall, I heard
him yelling that my slamming the door confirmed everything he
thought about me.

I was completely shaken by this episode, and, while I know
that this man was not representative of the profession, it ended
my willingness to look for help in that direction. I think this
episode is also illustrative, albeit in a very extreme way, of that
box I referred to earlier. If you have a view of the world, it is all
too easy to see everything as supporting it. It also occurred to
me at the time that had I been suicidal or emotionally vulnerable, that episode might well have been the last straw. I do
imagine that what happened to me with that man was anomalous, and it has never made much sense to me. But it does serve
as an extreme example of what can happen to someone in the
position I was in at that time.

Perversely perhaps, instead of shaking my confidence in myself, that man convinced me that I had been right all along. Moreover, out of that experience, I found the strength to say, "No more." It did nothing to ease the difficulty of being sick for no "good reason," but it did affirm my belief in my own understanding of what was going on. I regained my certainty, which had been battered and diminished in the preceding years, that my perceptions of my own experience were, if not completely accurate, clearer than anyone else's. It also reinforced for me the notion (this is much clearer in retrospect) that my sense of integrity was in my own hands and I had to maintain it even if, in the end, I was the only one who believed in it. This episode, while bizarre in the extreme, had much value for me.

There were many times when I doubted myself. As I had gained a reputation for walking into walls, so did I become known for inexplicable bouts of weakness. People tended to joke about that and especially about my clumsiness. I was known as a klutz. My reluctance to talk to anyone—much less doctors—about physical problems increased. I began to dread (and expect) that phrase, "It's all in your head."

The very simple fact that I was not trusted and others were to say what was or was not going on with me was enormously important. That fact, combined with that phrase always lurking in the background, evoked an uncertainty in me that was profound. My sense of certainty and conviction in my own integrity was forever being tested against the way I knew others saw me. And could I really ignore the possibility that I was simply neurotic? This had happened to me twice; there was a significant cumulative impact both on me and on those who knew me.

There is nothing more important to me than trust and acceptance. Without them any relationship is fatally flawed. And during those years in most of my relationships, those essential qualities were in question. I've never thought that trust or acceptance is divisible. If trust is lacking on one issue, its existence on another is, for me, doubtful.

Once again, I slowly recovered and my strength returned. I went back to work as a paralegal, and Nick and I married and moved to Washington. A few years later we divorced; we remained extremely close and the best of friends to each other. I mention that divorce only because I think it important to say that my disease had nothing to do with it. Anecdotal evidence abounds about the high incidence of divorce associated with chronic disease. If anything, my disease strengthened our relationship.

For the next few years, I was basically fine. I tired easily and seemed to have a harder time than was quite normal with ordinary things like colds and flu. My recovery from injuries received in an automobile accident was prolonged, but by that time I was beginning to accept that that was the way I was. I could no longer tolerate heat at all, which, living in Washington, is not very convenient. My reputation for weakness and general unreliability increased.

In the year before I was finally diagnosed as having multiple sclerosis, I had been getting progressively weaker, having more and more difficulty walking, and over time experiencing many sensory symptoms—pins and needles, numbness, tingling, areas of solidity. "Areas of solidity" probably conveys little; it is difficult to describe but involves a small area, usually in an arm or leg, that feels solid, unchanging. During this time, I also received a new nickname from the people in my office, "Limpy," a name used with affection.

My difficulty walking became so extreme that I gave in and went to a doctor, a new one. I did not, because I simply could not bring myself to, tell him any of my history. And yet even without that, there was a very quick judgment made that it was "all in your head." He said, "Well, there isn't anything wrong with you. If you insist, there is a faint possibility you have arthritis. But there's nothing to be done for you." My heart sank. I had a vision of history repeating itself and I simply could not face it. And yet I was having more and more difficulty doing what needed to be done on a daily basis.

Being once again faced with being told I was merely depressed was extremely distressing and frustrating. I knew there was something wrong with my body, that I was not depressed. As time went by and I received no confirmation of this, I found the situation more and more depressing and the label of depression thus once again received some validation. I began to feel very hopeless.

At that time I was living with a friend whose notion of sharing was an absolute 50–50 division. I like that theory but firmly believe that in practice the percentages both do and must shift from time to time. We took turns getting the Sunday paper, a fairly short walk. One Sunday when it was my turn, there was two to three feet of unplowed snow on the ground. I said I couldn't get the paper that day as it was so difficult for me to walk. Well, in the end and because the Sunday paper is one of those things I find essential, I did go for that walk. It took me forever, and coming back I fell and didn't think I could get up. I remember lying in the snow and crying out of frustration and a sense of helplessness. When I finally struggled back, there was not only no sympathy (which I can live without) but it was clear that I was thought to be manipulative and a complainer, attempting to use my "weakness" as a way to get out of things that I didn't want to do.

I found then, and I still do, both of those judgments very hard to bear. I have never been a complainer and I go out of my way not to be manipulative. In fact, I think I probably go to extremes in an attempt to be honest. Yet during those years when there was no accepted and legitimate reason for my weakness, I was continually being seen as both a complainer and as manipulative. I found the knowledge that others so perceived me to be almost beyond bearing.

I remember once being asked by a close family member to baby-sit so he and the child's mother could go out together. I said I was sorry but I couldn't. I was feeling terribly weak and shaky; the thought of taking care of a four-year-old was overwhelming at that moment. The response was, "Oh, come on. There's nothing wrong with you. You just don't want to do it." I have never forgotten how I felt at that moment. Despair is the word that comes closest to describing my feelings. In the end, I did baby-sit; I was shamed into doing it, and, in retrospect, I am ashamed that I had not at that moment the courage (or more likely, the strength) to insist on the reality of my weakness. Instead, I gave in to another's interpretation of my condition.

One aspect of this complex was that any lack of participation on my part was seen as a social statement or a social strategy, as reflecting a desire not to participate. There was no acknowledgment or awareness that my lack of participation reflected purely and simply a physical limitation. I was continually set against others' definition of what I should do and be; what I was, because it lacked legitimacy, was not considered.

All those years I was struggling with something that others could not see at all and that I saw only dimly. Others, seeing the struggle, concluded that I was wrestling with a phantom. Hence the label of neurosis. My certainty that there was a physical reality at issue ebbed and flowed. I never entirely lost it but I came quite close. I was left with the sense that my integrity, even my self, depended on believing in my own perceptions and, at the least, not defining myself as I was defined by others. Of course, that is true for us all.

Finding myself again in the position I had been in twice before and having no real reason to believe that the outcome would be any different, I buried my head in the sand and hoped it would all go away. (I did buy a book on arthritis but it seemed to have no relation to what was happening to me.) As had happened before, however, it became more and more difficult for me to function. I became ever more convinced that there was something seriously wrong with me.

Eventually, a friend recommended a new doctor and I pulled together what was left of my courage and saw him. He took one look at me and said that I clearly did not have arthritis. He listened carefully and this time I did relate my history. He won my confidence and my undying devotion by quickly saying that I clearly was not normal and there was something wrong. He referred me to a neurologist, who fairly quickly diagnosed multiple sclerosis.

After all those years there was an answer. The importance of competent medical care is clear. Doctors who listen carefully are rare. But I don't think necessarily that my doctors of earlier years were incompetent. My experience was not unique. At the best of times, multiple sclerosis is a difficult disease to diagnose with accuracy. It is easier and more certain now than it was fifteen years ago. I think what happened to me is much less likely to happen now. There is still no one definitive diagnostic test, but the advent of CT scanners, magnetic resonance imaging, and sophisticated evoked potential testing has certainly made diagnosis easier. Notwithstanding modern technology, however, many of the symptoms associated with multiple sclerosis, especially such inchoate things as fatigue and weakness, can be indicative of many diseases including depression. A good doctor is essential.

Since that time, five years ago, I have had several very difficult periods which my neurologist refers to as reintensifications. All of the symptoms I have ever had return in full force, but there is apparently no new disease activity. I have not had an acute exacerbation. At my best, I am almost "normal," although even then, my left leg is never entirely reliable. What I have learned is how very little it takes to upset the status quo. If I have a cold, or a fever, get overtired (which happens all too easily these days), or experience any kind of stress, my symptoms intensify. Summer in Washington is always a very bad time for me. Heat and humidity invariably result in a reappearance and worsening of symptoms. For example, under extreme stress—heat or fatigue—my speech difficulty recurs and my vision tends to blur.

I have, with time, learned ways of managing. Rest is usually the only way to get back to "normal," but because sick leave is a very limited commodity, rest can be difficult to get. I often find myself using weekends to recover from the week past and get ready for the one to come.

The question of legitimacy with a disease such as multiple sclerosis is never completely resolved. One's condition is not usually or necessarily reflected in one's appearance. And I found that receiving a diagnosis catapulted me from one world of perceptions and judgments to another—the world of being "sick." A different world now that my "sickness" was legitimate; nonetheless, another world and the central issue of maintaining my integrity remained.

The diagnosis of multiple sclerosis was for me a watershed— one of those events that radically transforms experience both past and future. It illuminated what had gone before and changed the terms of what was to follow. As an event, the diagnosis itself had limited meaning; it did not change my physical reality. Its importance lay in its power to transform the past, present, and future. The power of a name to alter reality is enormous.

The metaphorical power of the scene at the airport in Luxor comes alive for me through the prism of the diagnosis. Society, both before and after I received a diagnosis, shaped my experience. I was subject to other people's interpretation and judgment of my experience. People do tend to interpret reality through their own experience and view of the world and leave little room for others' worlds and other experiences of reality. For me, the primary goal was always to maintain my integrity within that interpretation. One way to do that, of course, and important in itself, is to step out of others' worlds. There is always an empty seat, as in Luxor, where one can sit and enjoy the scene.

# Multiple Sclerosis: The Disease

*In summary, MS is an unpredictable disease of the*
*nervous system which manifests primarily by disorders*
*in mobility. It is associated with a variety of other primary*
*and secondary symptoms and complications.*
*In general it is compatible with a long and productive life.*
LABE SCHEINBERG

What is multiple sclerosis? Over the years after my diagnosis I slowly formed a picture and gained some understanding of the disease. The name itself is revealing: multiple, more than one, and sclerosis, which refers to areas of sclerotic (scarred) tissue. Multiple sclerosis is a demyelinating disease of the white matter of the central nervous system.

These areas of sclerosis, also referred to as lesions or plaques, occur in the white matter of the central nervous system. Gray matter consists primarily of nerve cells. Axons (nerve fibers) are the connections between the cell body and the muscles, sensory organs, and primary organs such as the heart. These nerve cells are the communication system both within the central nervous system and between it and the rest of the body. Axons are sheathed in myelin, a white substance (hence the term "white matter") that insulates them and speeds transmission of impulses along the cell fibers. Electrical impulses move along the nerve fiber to the synapse (the connection point between cells) to the next nerve cell.

The lesions or plaques of multiple sclerosis are areas of tissue damage arising from inflammation, which occurs when white blood cells and fluid accumulate around blood vessels. This inflammation causes destruction of myelin. After the fragments are cleared away, a scar is formed—the lesion—in the area of demyelinization. The cause-and-effect process of inflammation and demyelinization is unclear. These lesions impede conduc-

16

tion of signals by blocking or slowing communication, either completely or partially and from time to time. The process can be thought of as similar to an electrical shortcircuit. The symptoms of multiple sclerosis result from that loss or diminution of signal conduction.

MS is the most common demyelinating disease of the central nervous system. In the United States alone, there are at least 250,000 cases. For reasons that remain unclear, it is more prevalent in northern temperate zones and affects noticeably more women than men. The average age of onset is thirty years.

Research into the underlying causes and processes of MS is ongoing, and in recent years, advances in virology and immunology have rapidly increased knowledge and understanding of the disease. However, its etiology remains unclear. Epidemiological studies indicate that an environmental factor, perhaps exposure to a virus, when combined with a genetic predisposition to the disease, may well control occurrence of the disease. MS is not a genetically transmitted disease. MS may also be or involve a defect of some kind in the body's autoimmune system—some part of the body may, in effect, attack itself.

Diagnosis of MS is difficult. A medical history and clinical examination must show at least two separate lesions that have occurred at more than one time. Obviously, any other possible causes must be ruled out. Because of the difficulty of diagnosis, the presence of MS is usually deemed to be either definite, probable, or possible. There is no one specific diagnostic test that can either confirm or rule out its presence.

A neurological examination can indicate lesions through the presence or absence of various signs and reflexes. A sign is an abnormality detected through examination, while a symptom is a subjective complaint noted by the patient. There is not necessarily a correlation between symptoms and signs. Signs may confirm symptoms or they may be asymptomatic. Symptoms may exist in the absence of signs.

Computerized tomographic (CT) scans will show some lesions. Magnetic resonance imaging usually reveals many more lesions than the CT scan, including some that may be subclinical, that is, they are not detectable through examination and may have no associated symptoms. An autopsy will usually show many more lesions than were ever suggested by either symptoms or signs. These lesions are probably the result of subclinical attacks of the disease.

Computerized testing of evoked potentials tests the brain's electrical responses to various forms of stimulation of the eyes, ears, or other parts of the body. Delays in these responses may indicate lesions that are clinically silent (producing no symptoms) and can sometimes firm up a questionable diagnosis from probable to definite MS. Testing of the cerebrospinal fluid for protein content, the number and type of white blood cells, and the amount of Ig6, a gamma globulin, can also support a diagnosis.

Symptoms of MS vary enormously, both from patient to patient and, over time, in one patient. Symptoms may include tingling, pins and needles, numbness, double or blurred vision, clumsiness of fine movements or of walking, frequency and urgency of urination, muscle weakness and spasms, pain or paralysis, incoordination, and mood or thought disturbances. According to one source, "Gait disorders varying from an inability to walk the usual distance to an inability to walk at all are the principal problems of patients with MS."[1]

Motor symptoms include weakness, spasticity, ataxia (loss of balance or incoordination), and speech disorders. Sensory symptoms include pins and needles, tingling, feelings of tightness or solidity (paresthesias), and, sometimes, sharp pains. Visual symptoms include blurred or double vision, nystagmus (involuntary eye movements), and, on occasion, blindness, which is almost always temporary. Urinary symptoms are common, as are frequent urinary tract infections. Energy problems include a lack of energy, easy fatiguability, and lack of endurance, particularly in the presence of heat and humidity.

Heat and humidity can be a real problem for those with MS, as mentioned earlier. Damaged nerve fibers have a strongly di-

---

1. Labe C. Scheinberg, "Signs, Symptoms, and Course of the Disease," in Labe C. Scheinberg, M.D., ed., *Multiple Sclerosis: A Guide for Patients and Their Families* (New York: Raven Press, 1983), p. 37.

minished tolerance for heat. Increases as little as 0.1° centigrade can decrease conduction or cause blockage, which will result in the appearance of symptoms.

The presence and effects of fatigue can be exceedingly difficult to live with and the fatigue of MS is often misunderstood. That phrase "It's all in your head" is all too easily applied to those who complain of fatigue. And I imagine everyone with MS has heard over and over, "But you look so good," usually accompanied by an expression, however slight, of incredulity. The fatigue of MS is special, and has several causes. Demyelinated nerve fibers use more energy to conduct impulses and thus fatigue more easily than normal fibers. Muscles that have been weakened result in a reliance on stronger muscles, which then tire faster. One recent report indicates that for those with MS the energy cost of walking is two to three times that of a normal person over the same distance.[2] Such an increased use of energy obviously results in increased fatigue.

The following is a good description of the fatigue associated with MS: "It involves large numbers of nerve fibers in a state of borderline function, which suddenly turn off when the body temperature is elevated only one or two degrees."[3] The signals suddenly cease to be transmitted, and one has to stop. The fatigue of MS is hard to describe. Sometimes when I go for a walk, I start out fine and after a block or two have a slight limp. As I continue to walk, my left leg begins to drag and hit the sidewalk. And then, sometimes very suddenly, I simply have to stop—the legs stop working. The exercise of will has nothing to do with it.

The course of the disease varies from one person to another and, like symptoms, may vary over time in the same person. There are three primary courses the disease may take: a benign course, involving a few early mild attacks followed by almost complete remission, leaving little or no disability; an exacerbating- remitting course with more early attacks with less complete remission resulting in some disability, followed by long periods

2. *Multiple Sclerosis Research Reports* 1, no. 2 (1987): 6.
3. Mark Wayland, "But You Look So Good," *Inside MS* 1, no. 4 (Fall 1983): 17.

of stability; and a progressive course involving a slow and continuing progression of the disease with no remission.

Some of those with an exacerbating-remitting course will eventually develop a slow progression involving fewer and less complete remissions with cumulative disabilities. Very rarely, there is a rapidly progressive course leading to death. MS itself is almost never the cause of death; death results from accompanying complications or infections. Generally speaking, the life expectancy of those with MS is at least 75 percent of normal.

Estimates of the percentage of cases in each group vary. The figures I have seen most often indicate that of the two-thirds of MS patients with an initially exacerbating-remitting course, 60 percent will eventually develop a slow progressive course. The other 40 percent will have a benign course. One-third of all patients show a slow progression from the beginning.

Exacerbations and remissions are difficult to define. The best definitions I have seen are these: exacerbation is "an acute appearance of new symptoms or worsening of old symptoms which lasts at least 24 hours," and remission is "a total or more often partial clearing of symptoms and signs which last[s] more than 24 hours."[4]

Symptoms may appear very rapidly, within minutes or days, or very slowly, over a period of weeks. They may be very transient and come and go rapidly. New symptoms may accumulate; old symptoms may reappear and/or intensify. My neurologist has taught me to look for persistence and duration in symptoms, and I try to be reasonably nonchalant about those that are fleeting in appearance.

Exacerbations—episodes of new disease activity—are not easy to diagnose with certainty. New symptoms may result from old, not new, areas of disease that were previously silent. Conversely, recurrence of old symptoms is not a sure indication of lack of exacerbation. Over time, the disease process may result in the formation of new plaques or the enlargement of existing ones. Again, there are varying figures available but one source indicates that only one-fifth of patients have new symptoms in

4. Scheinberg, *Multiple Sclerosis*, p. 42.

exacerbations; four of five have a recurrence of old symptoms.[5] Exacerbations can be caused by heat, physical trauma, extreme fatigue, psychological stress, infections, or any other kind of stress. While all of these factors have been associated with exacerbations, there is little empirical data to support these associations.

There does seem to be a direct correlation between the degree of remission from an exacerbation and its duration. For example, 85 percent will usually improve spontaneously from an exacerbation that lasts one week, but only 7 percent will improve after an exacerbation lasting one to two years. Over time, a series of exacerbations and remissions may result in a gradual accumulation of irreversible changes and disability.

There are factors that may be predictive of the course of the disease. An earlier age at onset may mean a more benign course. If, at onset, symptoms are sensory, the course of the disease may be less severe, while motor symptoms (weakness or incoordination) at onset may be predictive of greater disability. But again, as with everything to do with this disease, variation is extreme and the course and progression of the disease is unpredictable.

There is no cure for multiple sclerosis. Many promising modes of treatment are being developed and tested but most remain experimental. The commonly available treatments are essentially palliative. One drug which has been shown to shorten the duration and intensity of acute exacerbations is adrenocorticotropic hormone (ACTH), a pituitary gland substance that stimulates the adrenal glands to produce additional cortisone, which acts to reduce the inflammation in the brain or spinal cord. ACTH does not affect the underlying disease processes but may diminish the frequency and severity of exacerbations and even slow the progression of the disease.[6]

New drugs and new treatments are continually being developed. Recent press reports about a new experimental drug, Cop 1, are very promising. Preliminary results indicate that the drug

5. Ibid, pp. 31–32.
6. *Therapeutic Claims in Multiple Sclerosis* (New York: National Multiple Sclerosis Society, 1986), p. 105.

may slow and even reverse myelin destruction in those at an early stage of a benign form of multiple sclerosis.[7] It is important to remember, however, that promising early experimental results have often been reported and then later shown to be essentially useless. An enormous amount of research is currently being done on the causes and processes of multiple sclerosis, and understanding of the disease continues to increase.[8]

The most important fact about multiple sclerosis is its unpredictability and its uncertainty. There are very few certainties to be found anywhere in any aspect of this disease.

7. "Drug Slows Mild Multiple Sclerosis," *New York Times*, 13 August 1987, p. A19; "Multiple Sclerosis Drug Promising, Researchers Say," *The Washington Post*, 13 August 1987, p. A23.

8. Other sources which have been useful in forming my understanding of MS include: Byron H. Waksman and William E. Reynolds, *Research on Multiple Sclerosis* (New York: National Multiple Sclerosis Society, 1982); P. J. Vinken and G. W. Bruyn, eds., *Handbook of Clinical Neurology*, vol. 9 (New York: American Elsevier Publishing Company, 1971); Douglas McAlpine, Charles E. Lumsden, and E. D. Acheson, *Multiple Sclerosis: A Reappraisal*, 2d ed. (Baltimore: Williams and Wilkins, 1972); Bryan Matthews, *Multiple Sclerosis: The Facts* (Oxford: Oxford University Press, 1978); and J. F. Hallpike, C. W. M. Adams, and W. W. Tourtellotte, eds., *Multiple Sclerosis, Pathology, Diagnosis and Management* (Baltimore: Williams and Wilkins, 1983).

# Experience in Conflict with
# Received Wisdom

*. . . be still, and wait without hope*
*For hope would be hope for the wrong thing . . .*
T. S. ELIOT

My first reaction to receiving a diagnosis of multiple sclerosis was one of shock and terror, mixed with a deep sense of relief. I was stunned and I knew very little about the disease, which added to my terror, but at the same time there was overwhelming relief in knowing there was a solid physiological reason for the symptoms and inexplicable bouts of illness I had experienced over the years.

Receiving a diagnosis, any diagnosis, therefore, gave me a sense of great relief. I was not merely neurotic; there was a reason for what had happened to me over the years. I felt immensely vindicated and affirmed.

The way in which I learned of the diagnosis was responsible for much of my shock. My first inkling came as I stood before the counter in the radiology department of a large teaching hospital waiting to be checked in for a CT scan. As the nurse verified the information on the order form, I automatically read it upside down and saw in the diagnosis column, the words "multiple sclerosis." Staggering slightly and feeling as though I had been kicked in the stomach, I stumbled to a chair. I desperately tried to recall what I knew about multiple sclerosis. Very little, I realized—a neurological disorder, disabling—and what I did remember all seemed very devastating. My neurologist had carefully refrained from telling me what he thought might be wrong, saying that he wanted to wait until he was sure. I had gathered that something was wrong, and that it might be serious, but

23

somehow that didn't ease the shock of seeing those two words in print on the radiology order form.

I managed to get through the rest of that afternoon but my mind was reeling. Instead of going back to work I headed home, stopping at three bookstores on the way looking for a book on multiple sclerosis. I had to know exactly what this disease was and what its implications were before I could begin to think about it. Of course, there were no books to be found. I stopped at the library, but there were no books there either and I was too anxious and unsettled to sit in the reference room looking for information.

Once home I gathered together all the reference books in the house and began going through them. Some, but not much, information slowly emerged. Multiple sclerosis was a potentially progressive disease of the central nervous system, a demyelinating disease. Myelin—that rang a bell from anatomy courses. Slowly I began to form a picture of the disease.

Eventually I found many books, one of which I highly recommend to those newly diagnosed with multiple sclerosis and their families. *Multiple Sclerosis: The Facts* gives the facts, precisely, and presents a good overview of the disease and its possible implications.[1] The National Multiple Sclerosis Society is an excellent source of information about the disease, and its local chapters provide many services including counseling and support groups.[2]

The issues I found most problematic, however—the impact of MS on my sense of self and on my self-esteem; its effect on relationships; and the effects on me of the social construction of disease—were not discussed in what I read. A book has since been published, *The Body Silent* by Robert Murphy, which does address many of these issues.[3] Although it is not about multiple sclerosis, the issues remain the same.

1. Bryan Matthews, *Multiple Sclerosis: The Facts* (Oxford: Oxford University Press, 1978).

2. National Multiple Sclerosis Society, 205 East 42nd Street, New York, N.Y. 10017.

3. Robert Murphy, *The Body Silent* (New York: Henry Holt and Company, 1987).

The physical consequences of MS for me vary tremendously from day to day. As I mentioned, at the time of my diagnosis I was having considerable difficulty walking. My left leg was very weak and generally unreliable. My left arm felt quite dead and heavy, and it, too, was extremely weak. At the same time, I had a host of unpleasant sensations—tingling, numbness—all very hard to describe in a way that conveys much meaning to others. I had balance problems, was very weak, and tired extremely easily.

Over time, I have learned that there are good days and bad days in isolation as well as good and bad periods. There are times when every symptom I have ever had returns in full force (those periods of reintensification) and days when I feel almost (but never quite) "right." On a bad day I may have difficulty with balance, a hard time walking and especially climbing stairs, and quite severe weakness and fatigue. I sometimes feel as though I expend an enormous amount of energy merely having and dragging around my left side. These good and bad days often seem to be unrelated to anything in particular. At times these symptoms are clearly attributable either to extreme heat or cold or severe stress of one form or another.

Why do I feel another book on MS is necessary? There is certainly ample information available on the medical aspects of multiple sclerosis. Medical texts and journal articles were very helpful in forming my understanding of the disease. But, having read this literature, I was struck by its general lack of utility for the newly diagnosed and particularly for those fortunate enough to have a fairly benign form of the disease. More specifically, the literature generally fails to deal with the psychological process of adjustment to multiple sclerosis. In particular, the issues and questions that concern me, that have arisen out of and been clarified by my experience of the last few years, are not generally discussed.

Much of the literature is geared to those who are very ill or severely disabled. It fails to speak to those who may be quite "well" but who still have a significant adjustment to make. Most of the books and articles available do not deal with the initial reactions to learning that one has a chronic and potentially

disabling disease, the knowledge of which, however benign its
course, will radically affect one's life. The disease may be physically devastating, and one is forced to realize and accept all of
its possibilities—I may very well become completely physically
dependent on others. The emotional impact of multiple sclerosis
and the host of issues involved in coming to terms with the disease are generally glossed over lightly by most writers.

Many of the books on MS are personal stories of the "how to
live with multiple sclerosis" variety. I read these eagerly with
the hope that I, too, would learn how to live with multiple sclerosis. Most of these stories were interesting; some were moving.
They were not, however, particularly helpful to me at that time.
I was devastated by the awareness that I had a disease which
could irrevocably alter the course of my life. I needed acknowledgment of that fact, and I needed help in coming to terms with
it and moving beyond the despair I felt.

Instead, I found that most of these writers failed to acknowledge the emotional impact of receiving such a diagnosis. The
authors focused on the physical adjustments necessary to live
with their varying disabilities and limitations. This was useful
information but not what I immediately needed. I had no doubt
that with determination and care ways could be found to cope
with, and learn to live with, physical limitations. But before that
was possible I had to accept the deeper implications of a life
framed by the knowledge that I had a potentially crippling and
devastating disease.

A mundane but, for me, telling example involved the warnings I was given by my doctor to avoid heat, cold, stress of any
kind, exposure to colds or other viruses, and, it seemed, just
about all of the normal vicissitudes of daily life. On a purely
physical level, this is very clear and, I realized immediately,
equally impossible. Presumably, however, physical and practical responses to such advice were to be found. But there was
another side to this that was not addressed and for which I
found no answer. What are the psychological implications of
such warnings? When I first heard them, I was frightened and
unsure; under the surface were questions of responsibility and
control, the dynamics of daily life and relationships, the need to

fashion a life which was lived fully and normally and yet without either overreacting to these warnings or disregarding them
completely.

How does the knowledge that one has multiple sclerosis affect and change one's life? How should it? As I struggled through
the succession of issues that were raised for me, it would have
been very useful—not to mention comforting—to have known
what might be involved and how others in my position had reacted. Coming to terms with the fact of having a disease such as
MS would have been greatly eased and facilitated for me had
there been an acknowledgment and discussion of the process of
emotional and psychological adjustment. My responses might
not have changed but there is reassurance in knowing that one
is not unique. Some knowledge of the issues involved would
have eased the way.

Or was my response unique? I found it hard to believe that it
was and yet I could find no acknowledgment of the issues that,
even early on, were most difficult for me—the impact of the disease on my sense of self, my competence, my worth, and the
effects on those I was closest to and our relationships. This lack
of confirmation increased my difficulty; I wondered if I was
overreacting or if my responses were completely out of line with
the reality.

The varying reactions of friends and relatives to my diagnosis are examples of an issue that turned out to be significant and
*difficult for me but which I rarely saw mentioned in the books I*
read. Those reactions, while fascinating in and of themselves
and adding to my store of knowledge about people and relationships, were difficult to deal with; some warning of what might
be encountered would have been very helpful.

As I read these books, I realized that in addition to their failure to speak to my experience, they shared several common assumptions. These included the notion that adjustment to the
disease requires only a physical response, that hope and an optimistic outlook will conquer all obstacles and, therefore, that
failure to overcome the disease flows in large part from defects in character and will. I began to think there was a connection between these underlying—and not always explicit—

assumptions and the fact that what I was experiencing was not addressed. Perhaps it was the very fact of these assumptions that prevented discussion of the issues that were so central for me. Was it because of a common assumption, for example, that a failure to overcome obstacles reveals a defect in character that some of the obstacles and issues I felt were not mentioned? For to mention them, to acknowledge an unremovable obstacle, would be felt as revealing such a character deficit. Or, perhaps, dealing with MS on a purely physical level was a way of avoiding the necessary conclusion that one's very self is at issue and at stake in any real adjustment.

The implication that physical adjustment was all that was necessary to live with MS was very clear in most of what I read and conflicted strongly with what I was experiencing. I would not minimize the difficulty of walking with aids, or not walking at all, and the need to reorganize one's daily life around such eventualities, but it seemed to me then—and now—that such changes are secondary to an emotional and psychological accommodation to the *fact* of the disease. The physical fact of walking with difficulty is not nearly so important as the psychological and social consequences.

It also seemed that most of these writers used hope as a mask, a way of screening them from the full implications of acceptance. Part of my despair stemmed from the fact that there is no cure for multiple sclerosis and available treatments are merely palliative. I saw no way to avoid facing that reality, and it was only through full acceptance of its implications that I could move beyond despair.

Hope is a necessary component of living with the disease, as it is a necessary part of life. But hope is possible only after full acceptance of present reality and potential consequences. To use hope, either of change or improvement, as a barrier to complete realization of the potential consequences of multiple sclerosis seemed not only self-defeating but impossible. For me, hope could only come into play after acceptance. In most of what I read, however, it seemed that hope was pursued before acceptance was achieved. The language itself was very revealing: "pursuit of hope," "quest for hope," "find hope," "fought and conquered the fear, uncertainty and despair" of MS. Hope was used as a weapon. For me, hope is important but it comes into play only within the parameters of experienced reality. And then, it is hope of living fully and with some integrity within the given context of my life.

It also became apparent that most of these authors felt that optimism was a requirement; that it was not acceptable to acknowledge the psychological pain they may have felt. Or if, in fact, they felt no pain, then what was wrong with me? Optimism, as with hope, if used to screen out reality, becomes an impediment to full acceptance, and, without that acceptance, a true optimism about life becomes impossible to achieve. The knowledge that one has a disease such as multiple sclerosis is in many ways unacceptable; nevertheless, acceptance is crucial. Hope and optimism as they were used in these stories seemed to obviate the need for acceptance, foreclose the need to deal with reality, and support denial. Or was it rather that denial led to hope? I began to wonder whether, in either case, hope used in this way did not foreclose discussion of the issues that seemed so important to me.

A third assumption that I began dimly to perceive was that failure in "living with MS," or acceptance of and giving in to the limits imposed by the disease, was seen by these authors as indicating weakness; that if one only tried hard enough, one could push the limits—giving in was not acceptable. The common response to a handicap of any kind is "try harder." The cultural emphasis on independence and individualism further complicates this issue.

I am aware of the psychological difficulty of asking for help, of saying "I'm sorry, I can do no more." It is difficult to be seen as not trying hard enough. Yet there are times when one can do no more, when one must give in, when the disease forces acceptance of physical limits. At those times, one must be able to give in to those facts, recognize those limits, without feeling guilty or weak.

There is clearly a very fine line between not trying hard enough and trying too hard. But achieving that balance is enormously complicated by an assumption that if one fails, it is necessarily because one has not tried hard enough. It is also

complicated by the uncertainty of MS and the daily changes
in strength and capacity that make it very difficult for either
oneself or others to have any consistently useful and straightforward idea of that capacity. To talk about "conquering" the
uncertainty of MS is to miss the point: MS is uncertain; one of
its foremost attributes is uncertainty.

During this time I only dimly perceived the issues raised for
me by the strength/weakness dilemma and its importance. Why
is it so hard to acknowledge weakness? Why did I feel that I had
to be strong to ask for help? Over the years as I began to resolve
the conflict for myself, I slowly became aware of the degree to
which this issue reflected a set of cultural values. It illuminated
some part of the conflict between self and culture and what it
means to be sick or disabled in this society.

I had become notorious within my family over the years for
failing to rake leaves. Our summer house is inundated every fall
by what seem to be millions and millions of leaves. I have always felt rather strongly that if God intended leaves to be raked,
he would have seen to it that rakes evolved as part of trees. Nevertheless, there is a strong feeling in my family that leaves must
be raked and moved and that full participation in this process
is a social requirement. I simply could not rake leaves for more
than a few minutes at a time. Standing and working is almost
impossible for me, and I garden on my hands and knees. My
weakness was ignored and I was openly seen and treated as a
shirker and a wimp. The feeling was clearly that I used my
"weakness" as an excuse to get out of a task I disliked.

Raking leaves became family shorthand for a whole set of
behavior that, while a result of my weakness and fatigue, was
seen by my family as shirking, getting out of unpleasant tasks,
and as a reflection of a lack of will, ultimately of character.
Given my history—that there was never anything "really" wrong
with me—this attitude had some justification. I was uncomfortable (and defensive to a degree) because my weakness had no
social reality or validity. When my MS was discovered, leaf raking was mentioned by all my family: "Aha, that's why she
couldn't rake leaves." And on that level there was some new
clarity. But to my dismay that clarity in relationships did not

reach very far and the effect on me of those years of being seen as a non-leaf-raker was longstanding.

My first reactions of terror and relief at the diagnosis of MS slowly faded, to be replaced by a kind of cloudiness. There were so many implications and they were so interrelated that it took a long time before they began to fall into place. There was the first cold after my diagnosis, when, remembering all those warnings, I anxiously waited for a relapse, which failed to materialize. And, on a more diffuse level, there was a dawning realization that all of my close relationships were affected. No relationship is static, but I felt as though a large rock had been thrown into the pool of each of my relationships; there were new currents, and a need to reform the patterns to accommodate this new fact.

I also began to see (and this is much clearer in retrospect) that both of my first emotions—terror and relief—were largely inappropriate. The terror was not lasting. I learned that I would survive, perhaps not as I would wish, but I could and did learn to live within the framework of chronic disease. The relief, however, was also false. I had really felt that receiving a diagnosis would make everything OK vis-à-vis other people. That once there was a defined, definite, and legitimate reason for my bouts of illness and my physical weakness over the years, that would be that. That once there was an explanation of my inability to rake leaves for hours, I would not be seen and treated as a shirker. This particular dilemma became a model for me of the critical aspects of adjustment. If I could more fully comprehend its parts, perhaps I could see more clearly the relationship between society and the individual in the context of chronic disease. It was deeply disappointing that not only was everything not OK, simple and discrete, but that, in fact, both close relationships and my relation to society in general became even more complicated and, at least initially, even more difficult.

Culturally legitimated expectations of disability and disease are very different. A handicap is seen as a stable condition and yet, curiously, one which should not be accepted—as reflected in the common admonition to try harder and never give in. Disease, on the other hand, is seen as having one of two possible outcomes—the patient will get better or he will die. Those with a relapsing-remitting form of MS, however, have a disease from which they will not recover but from which they will not die. They also may have disabilities which vary enormously in both their impact and their visibility from day to day. And, even at those times when they are most handicapped by the disease, they may look very well indeed. The common understandings of illness and disability and the role expectations associated with them are often confounded by MS.

Immediately after my diagnosis, when I was searching for certainty and answers to questions I had only dimly formulated, my response to the books on MS was one of discouragement. If the only way to live with multiple sclerosis was to avoid its reality and its potential consequences, to take refuge in hope—how could I begin to come to terms with the disease? My thoughts about hope and denial were primarily intuitive, and it was only much later that I began to think about the implications of the assumptions I found underlying most of what I read.

Over time, I began to think about the ways in which hope, for example, as it seemed to be used in what I read was tied in with the idea, so prevalent in this culture, that everything can be changed, everything can be fixed, and its corollary, that failure results from defects in character, intelligence, or will. I also began to wonder about the ways in which common understandings and reactions to disability and disease shape the responses of those who are ill or disabled, not just the reactions of others to them. The nature of MS perhaps further complicates this process because someone with MS may float in and out of disease and disability and have no fixed status. Was the denial I saw in these stories a reflection of the desire not to be cast into the sick/disabled role because of its negative connotations and consequences in this culture? To what degree were these assumptions culturally mandated? How deeply did culturally legitimated expectations of disability and illness shape and, indeed, distort individual experience?

What was clear to me at the time was that the help I needed was not available and that my need for help remained unacknowledged. Moreover, the assumptions and implicit understandings that I found reflected in the books I read not only provided no help, but were destructive and impeded the necessary process of emotional adjustment. Adjustment is necessary. The new knowledge of disease must be integrated into one's sense of self; the self must be re-formed around it. Continued life and growth is possible only through and after this adjustment. The fact of the disease must take its proper place so that one can be more than a person with MS.

Hope was not enough. Hope did not help me to understand and ultimately to accept and adjust to the impact of the disease on my primary relationships. Trying harder was no answer to the impact on my sense of worth and competence of knowing that my brain was damaged. Learning to live with the potential of dependency and how and when to ask for help was in no way made easier by the implication that failure to manage would arise out of defects in my will. Striving only to meet the ideal of independence and a stiff upper lip would have required that I deny the very real limits and changes imposed on me by the disease.

My first need was to achieve a realistic, tempered, and yet, within those limits, optimistic outlook on life. To do that I had to deal with the emotional and psychological issues raised for me by the fact of this disease. The process of adjusting to the fact of MS in my life was complex, long-lasting, and necessarily on-going.

At the time of my diagnosis I was, as much as anyone ever can be, in a fairly good position to receive such news. The circumstances of my life were rather straightforward. I was old enough to have a reasonably good idea of who I was, what was important, and what I believed. Hard as it was for me during all the years when I did not know what was wrong with me, I think that when I did receive a diagnosis it was easier to come to terms with the knowledge that I had a chronic disease than it might have been earlier.

My life was structurally rather simple. I was in my late thirties, divorced, and childless, and living in a community where I had been for some years and had some roots. I had a job I enjoyed and I was about to start graduate school in a subject I loved. But the facts of our lives convey very little about who we are; they seem to be not very relevant. They have little to do with the emotional and psychological issues that a disease such as MS brings to the fore. In their basic outline, these issues are the same for everyone.

I think, for me, the knowledge that I have MS has acted primarily as a great clarifier. It has changed me in some ways but mostly it accelerated the process of stripping down that I think usually occurs as we age. Most of my feelings about life have been reaffirmed. Many of the changes have been external. I found that I simply lacked the strength to work full-time and go to school and that, since work was essential, there was no choice but to leave graduate school. Another consequence of MS has been that I do now take work more seriously than I once did. I was never ambitious and never had or desired a career. Work for me was always a means to an end. Now it is not enough to say, "Well, I can always get a job and support myself." I am more concerned with financial and job security, pensions and benefits. After all those years, I tried to get myself into a position with some advancement possibilities. Work is still a means to an end but financial security is more important to me now, and achieving that requires a slightly more serious attitude about work than I once had.

But my beliefs about life, my thoughts about what is important, have not changed. I am not religious, although I was raised in the tradition of mainstream Christianity. Religion permeated my childhood and my rejection of it was not without thought. For me, religion is a means to avoid seeing clearly and to shelter oneself from reality. It seems to me that religion is often used as a cover for, even a promotion of, hypocritical and dishonest behavior. I think that most religious behavior obscures life and takes the edge off reality. Having MS has made me want to be even more clear about exactly what life is and to be direct in my response to it.

A disease such as MS exposes one to perhaps more than the usual amount of hypocrisy and dishonesty and dramatically decreases one's tolerance for such things. Because disease is so clarifying in many ways, one loses any remaining doubt about what really does matter and what really is worth fussing about. None of this is meant to suggest that I don't do my share and more of mistreating people and unnecessarily flailing around. But, at root, there is a new level of understanding about what is and is not important.

My sense of the ridiculous in people and life continues to increase and I would not like to have lived through the last few years without it. There are moments when I am full of despair but I generally am rescued by seeing the absurdity of it all. There was a day when I fell in front of my employer and he very carefully stepped over me and walked away without a word. That was a very funny scene. Laughing at myself and others, seeing how ridiculous we all can be, has been a central part of the last few years.

The meaning of life seems more and more to be a useless question. I have come to believe—and having a chronic disease has, if anything, intensified this—that searching for meaning, or even ascribing meaning, in many ways obscures meaning. I don't think there is much in the way of a grand purpose to be found in life. Life is a gift and what matters is to live honestly and without illusion, insofar as that is possible for any of us; to see what is and respond openly and wholeheartedly. And people matter—the care and attention with which we know and love one another.

As I have lived with this disease and all it means, I have come to think that I would like to live as a good gardener. Gardening involves clarity and honest appraisals; there is no room for games. The processes are very direct and clean. There is an abundance of laughter and joy to be found and no lack of mystery, but the mystery is not overlain with illusion.

Learning that I had multiple sclerosis was a shock. Coming to terms with it, and integrating that knowledge into my life and my sense of who I am, is a long and continuing process.

# After the Diagnosis

*I was told that . . . I might or might not experience
symptoms of neural damage all my life. These symptoms, which
might or might not appear, might or might not involve my eyes.
They might or might not be disabling. . . .*

JOAN DIDION

What happens after one is told one has a disease such as MS?
The diagnosis is made and, usually sooner rather than later, one
is thrown back into life and left alone to confront this new reality. It is a bit like learning to swim by being thrown in the
water. I felt as though I had been presented with a task that was
undefined and for which there were no guidelines.

My experience in coming to terms with the fact of multiple
sclerosis in my life has led me to believe that there are several
parts to the immediate and very personal process of acceptance.
There are the initial reactions to the diagnosis and how one
deals with them. There are the ways in which MS does and does
not affect daily life. There is the host of emotional issues raised
by the disease. Finally, there are the ways in which the very fact
of a disease such as MS affects relationships. These were all involved in my attempts both to come to terms with multiple sclerosis and to incorporate the reality of the disease into my life
without letting it dominate my life.

The first few months after the diagnosis were difficult for
me. Despite my neurologist's assurance that I had a relapsing-
remitting form of the disease, which was likely to be fairly benign, at least initially, I was convinced that the worst would
happen and happen rapidly. I think this reaction was probably
inevitable. It is also clear, with hindsight, that a primary task
for me was coming to see myself as mildly disabled and prone
to occasional bad spells but basically healthy; that would have

been much easier to achieve had I known more about the adjustment process. It was almost a year before I relaxed and stopped seeing impending disaster in every new sensation and symptom. It took time to learn the new parameters of normality.

One benefit of the diagnosis was learning that some very strange things that had happened to me over the years did, indeed, fall within these normal parameters. One is called Lehrmitte's syndrome—moving one's head in a certain way produces a sometimes severe sensation of electrical shock. The other is a sudden sensation of water pouring down the back of a leg. The feeling is so real in every way that I would reach down to touch my wet skirt and be amazed and unbelieving to find absolute dryness. These are not uncommon symptoms with MS, and it was very nice to be able to slot them into that disease complex. Over the years as I read about MS, I would come across descriptions of other symptoms and say, "Aha, that is what that was." These were not things I had ever mentioned to a doctor, either because they were transient, because I had forgotten them, or because they seemed so bizarre that I hesitated to mention them. Explanation even in retrospect is very comforting.

There are good days and there are bad days, and a bad day does not necessarily, or even usually, mean a recurrence of the disease. Recognizing how fatigue, heat, stress, and even a fever can affect symptoms and one's daily ability to function takes a long time. It takes even longer to learn to accept such daily changes with equanimity. There is a big difference between gaining an intellectual knowledge of the disease and living with it as a permanent and daily companion. I am still uneasy about recurrences but I no longer await them with trepidation, nor do I interpret every new or recurring symptom as representing a new onset of the disease.

Along with all the medical information and the constant reassurance I received from my neurologist, it would have been very helpful if I had had some notion of what was involved emotionally in coming to terms with multiple sclerosis. Particularly if one has a benign form of the disease and functions reasonably well, there seems to be an expectation that one will come to terms with it easily and quickly. In contrast, I think someone who is very ill and very disabled will be expected to have more difficulty and hence will receive much more overt emotional support. I could be wrong.

What I heard, however, particularly from medical professionals, was a version of "Yes, you have multiple sclerosis, but you are basically fine and, therefore, your life should not change nor should it be difficult to adapt to it." That is wrong. The knowledge that one has a potentially serious and debilitating disease—no matter how benign a form it seems to be taking— does change one's life and requires a significant adjustment. That knowledge is not easy to accept. Recognition of that reality by the medical profession would have provided a level of support that was missing for me. My adjustment might well have been easier and quicker. One can certainly overreact or make the disease the centerpiece of one's life, and I am by no means advocating that, but the difficulty of coming to terms with it should not be understated.

"Living with multiple sclerosis" or some version thereof seems, as I mentioned earlier, to be a popular title for books on the disease. There is good reason for this—it is the primary task of anyone who has the disease. One must live with multiple sclerosis; it will not go away. As Congressman Morris Udall said about Parkinson's disease, "I won't die *from* it, but I will die *with* it."[1] Having MS does not have to become the predominant reality of life, although when first diagnosed it can be very difficult to think otherwise. Recognizing the ways in which the disease does impinge on one's life and making the necessary adjustments, physical or emotional, are first steps toward identifying the areas in which the disease need not be a factor. The knowledge that one has multiple sclerosis does change one irrevocably and significantly, but it is possible to see one's self as a person who has multiple sclerosis rather than as a "multiple sclerosis person" (an unfortunate term I have seen used from time to time).

Learning to view oneself as a healthy person who has a

1. Quoted in Myra MacPherson, "Mo Udall, Triumph of the Good Guy," *Washington Post*, 29 December 1985, p. K5.

chronic disease—paradoxical, perhaps, but nonetheless true—takes time. It also requires, of course, that one have a relapsing-remitting form of the disease and be reasonably free of symptoms most of the time. I was fairly free of symptoms but immediately after my diagnosis I thought of myself as sick, which, of course, affected my outlook on life enormously. I found it almost impossible to forget for a moment that I had multiple sclerosis and I allowed it to take over my life. I was, during that time, a "multiple sclerosis person." It mattered not a whit what the doctors said—I could not be reassured.

Over the course of the next year, reassured mainly by the passage of time, I began to see myself as an otherwise healthy person with an underlying but, for the most part, inactive disease. There were, however, some significant ways in which the disease affected my daily life that demanded attention and readjustment. The primary task was learning to live with day to day uncertainty.

There is uncertainty in all of life; events occur over which one has no control and of which one has no warning. The uncertainty of multiple sclerosis is of a different order, however. It is both more urgent and more threatening because it emanates from a very real, ever-present cause and it cannot be ignored. There is the uncertainty of the future—what will happen to me, will I be able to walk in five years, ten years? These are not frivolous questions. It is likely that the disease will recur at some time. Then there is the more immediate uncertainty of tomorrow—will I be able to walk those ten blocks to do that errand I have planned? Uncertainty about the future will not go away, although one can learn over time to come to terms with it.

Long-term uncertainty becomes easier to accept once some accommodation with daily uncertainty has been reached, partly because it is no longer quite so easy to deny the possibilities of the future. But this does require fully integrating the facts and all the implications of the disease into one's view of self. It involves accepting the potential of physical dependency, something that was and remains very hard for me. Part of my horror came from even contemplating the possibility that I might become physically dependent on others. I had to come to terms with my fear before I could view the future—or even the present—with any equanimity. Some people say, "You may never become physically dependent, therefore don't worry about it." For me, it was necessary to reach some psychological accommodation with the possibilities so they could be put in perspective. Having achieved some degree of acceptance of what might happen to me, I can be less at the mercy of my fear.

Uncertainty about tomorrow requires more immediate adjustment. It is easy to feel anger and frustration when, because one's physical capacity varies so from day to day, plans cannot always be carried out. It becomes even more necessary than usual to know one's priorities. The need to establish priorities is common to everyone but becomes more acute under the pressure of this level of daily uncertainty. I also discovered that my expectations of what I should be capable of were getting in my way. I had to learn to adjust those expectations to the reality of what I was capable of and, more important, to understand that who I was did not depend on what I could do physically. I found that I was concerned about what others would think of me—a self-created difficulty; others usually respected my limits once they were made aware of them. It was hard for me to recognize my limits (especially because they changed so from day to day), but when I did, and conveyed them directly to others, much of my difficulty disappeared. There are, of course, those who will never respect my limits and, in the end, I simply have to accept that.

While reading about marathon runners, I came across the phrase "wall of fatigue." I was delighted to find it because it expressed so perfectly the degree of fatigue I sometimes felt and had extraordinary difficulty in describing to others. Since then, an article on fatigue, "But You *Look* So Good," has appeared in a National Multiple Sclerosis Society publication.[2] "Looking so good" is exactly what makes dealing with fatigue in multiple sclerosis so difficult. I look young, energetic, and healthy and it can be very difficult to explain to an employer, for example, that

2. Mark Wayland, "But You Look So Good," *Inside MS* 1, no. 4 (Fall 1983): 16–17.

there are times when walking across a room seems impossible. The onset of this fatigue can be totally unpredictable and, even to those who know one very well, imperceptible. When the article appeared, I gave a copy to my employer. He became more understanding and our daily relations were much easier for both of us. I felt freer to acknowledge those times when fatigue was a real problem and he became more sensitive to my needs. But he had to be made aware of those needs and that was up to me. I have had to remember that explanation (as, for example, when I change jobs) continues to be necessary.

It is very difficult for me to admit that I am tired—to others or myself. And once again, it is important to realize that generally it is one's own expectations that are at stake. It was hard for me to learn that people would not think less of me when I admitted that I was too tired to make dinner, go to the movies, or sit up late and talk. It was difficult to admit that I could not always do everything I had planned. And that "wall of fatigue" can be encountered at very inconvenient times. Once I learned to admit to myself that I could not always do what I wanted when I wanted, I found that others were usually very understanding. But I had to learn to be direct and honest with the people involved. More important, I had to learn to accept that there was a basic uncertainty about my day-to-day life that was not within my control.

Asking for help was not easy for me. I have always been fairly independent and self-sufficient. Suddenly there were times when I was not able to do things I had always taken for granted— small things usually, but important to me. Asking for a ride home from work or a hand carrying groceries was hard for me but I found that help, if asked for, was available and friends seemed pleased to assist. Once again, the resistance was mine. When I realized that no one thought less of me for admitting that I needed help and, more important, that there was no need for me to think less of me, that difficulty vanished.

The notion of responsibility also required attention. There was a need to sort out the ways in which I can take responsibility for my own well-being from those areas over which I have no control. Careful attention to diet, exercise, and rest, for example, can have an enormous effect on my day-to-day well-being and are entirely within my control. The underlying fact of the disease, however, is outside my control. I had some difficulty at first with the notion of responsibility because of the very nature of multiple sclerosis. It is perfectly possible to do all the right things, exercise, eat properly, avoid stress, and so on, and have a recurrence of the disease. It is also perfectly possible to do all the wrong things and not have a recurrence. The relationship between stress factors and recurrences is imperfectly understood, as mentioned earlier.

I still have difficulty with the whole idea of stress. The periods of reintensification I have experienced regularly over the years since my diagnosis can be very frustrating. Now that I understand such episodes better, I usually try to wait them out but occasionally I give up and resort to seeing my doctor. If he rules out some common causes—a urinary tract infection, a virus, a heat wave—his answer is usually that I must be under some psychological stress and there is nothing he can do about that. I never doubt that he is correct in his assessment, but I do find it difficult to deal with. Life is stressful, after all, and what produces stress varies enormously from person to person and from time to time. Much of what I find most stressful is not easily within my power to change. So I am left with the knowledge that it is my own response to the world that is creating the difficulty and that the only thing I can do about it is to try to change that response. Some well-intentioned people have suggested to me from time to time that the course of the disease is entirely within my control and that if I have a recurrence, it will be my fault. No, it will not be my fault, but it is important to recognize those things that are within my control and to take responsibility for them.

Most of these issues involved learning my limits, reordering my priorities, and communicating my needs and limits directly and honestly to my friends and colleagues. The difficulties I had on this level were to a large degree self-created. Either I failed to accept the changes in me and how they affected my behavior or I failed to communicate those changes to others. In retrospect, I think this process would have been much easier if I had had some awareness that these issues would, in fact, be issues.

Having discussed some of the practical difficulties in adjusting to multiple sclerosis, I come to the heart of what I see as central to acceptance and adjustment—the ways in which a disease such as multiple sclerosis forces one to come to terms with some very basic emotional issues. These issues are not dissimilar to those faced by all individuals and, in fact, some are the same. But they are heightened by having multiple sclerosis and have a greater degree of urgency. I also found that many emotional issues that I had previously confronted and resolved were once again open questions. I seemed, to some extent, to have been thrown back to an earlier stage of development and suddenly had to work through these issues again in light of the new realities of my life and to try to achieve new resolution of them.

Out of my own experience I have identified some areas in which the knowledge of having a disease such as multiple sclerosis has significant emotional impact. I firmly believe that each requires a certain amount of awareness and attention before the disease can be thoroughly integrated into one's life. Coming to terms with these issues is both necessary and solitary, but, again, knowledge of what may be involved can be helpful. For some, support groups may be an important resource. For others, it is by necessity or choice an individual process and for those people there is a dearth of information about what to expect. My intention here is not to engage in pseudo-psychologizing or to suggest answers but merely to indicate what the process of full acceptance of the disease may involve and some issues which may be encountered along the way.

The first issue—first because I believe it is at the heart of all the others and must be dealt with before the others can even be identified—is how severely the fact of the disease may affect one's self-image and even self-esteem. I don't think this is generally acknowledged as a difficulty for most of those with a reasonably benign form of multiple sclerosis, partly because there may be no objective change in outward appearance and partly because of a lack of sensitivity to how significant an effect minor physical changes may have on one's sense of self.

I have no idea how general my experience may have been but I do think that to some degree it is shared by all those newly diagnosed with multiple sclerosis. My diagnosis, while welcome in many ways, came, of course, at an awkward time for me. It would be hard to think of a convenient moment for such news. I was feeling very good about my life. I had a new job and I was about to begin graduate school. I was very excited and confident and that confidence had been hard won. It would have been very helpful if someone had taken the time to try to tell me some of what I was facing. I might have denied that I would react that way, but at least I would have known that coming to terms with multiple sclerosis involved more than purely physical adjustment.

It was not until I started graduate school—about two weeks after receiving the diagnosis—that I really began to see what had happened to my self-image and how that was affecting my behavior. My intellectual ability was not in question, and I had always enjoyed the give-and-take of classroom discussion. Yet suddenly I dreaded classes, tried to disappear in the back of the room, and was totally incapable of speaking up. My confidence was shattered, intellectually and socially. As I began to wonder why and to try to regain some assurance, I realized that I felt damaged and that this was affecting my entire approach to the world. I felt that all of me was damaged, including my mind, and I also had a sense that this was apparent to those around me. I had to force myself to attend class and especially to participate in discussion. Forcibly reminding myself over and over that, while I felt "damaged," my intellectual capacity was intact (or so I hoped), I slowly regained some confidence. I found that while I was avoiding some things, I was also putting myself in situations where my competence would be tested and reaffirmed. Regaining my confidence was a very slow process and involved learning to limit my sense of disability and damage to those physical changes that were objectively real.

Another example of how my feeling of disability affected me involved walking. I had always walked very quickly but over the year before my diagnosis, walking difficulties had become an almost daily occurrence. Even on the best days I walked fairly slowly and carefully, and on particularly bad days I crept along and was unable to cross the street before the light changed. Given that I appeared to be perfectly healthy, it is perhaps understandable that drivers honked and yelled at me and pedestrians stared. I, however, found it almost unbearable and it added to my sense of inadequacy and loss of control. It increased my sense of damage and disability because that disability was visible and was being visibly reacted to by others.

Walking slowly is one of life's more unimportant aspects but one that can take on a great deal of significance. I soon learned that if I waited until the beginning of the walk cycle, I could usually make it across the street and I became used to being stared at, although it is not something I am reconciled to and I tend to wear dark glasses excessively. And there was one advantage that I finally noticed, to my great delight—I had time to look closely at people walking toward me, more time to notice my surroundings, more time to observe those little bits of beauty that I had usually overlooked. But the fact remains that my difficulty walking, while not objectively great, had an extraordinary effect on me and it was not primarily physical.

I am convinced that the blows to and the changes in self-image and self-esteem are of primary importance in the process of adjustment to chronic disease and/or disability. Failure to acknowledge both these effects and their centrality makes true adjustment impossible. Curiously, there is a strong disinclination on the part of many, both disabled and non-disabled, to acknowledge this. In a review of Robert Murphy's wonderful book *The Body Silent,* which stresses the effects of disability on self-image and self-esteem, the reviewer states, Murphy "resorts to a painfully familiar response to social injustice—blaming the victim. He sees a negative self-image as the inevitable fate of disabled persons."[3]

Self-esteem *is* a primary issue for those confronted with chronic illness and disability. Yet this reviewer, a psychotherapist and herself disabled, calls this point of view "damaging and unfounded" and goes on to say that disability is a social, not an individual, problem. Of course, disability exists for the indi-

3. Harilyn Rousso, "Witness to Life: A Quadriplegic's Journey," review of Robert F. Murphy, *The Body Silent, Washington Post Book World,* 29 March 1987, p. 9.

vidual in a social context and its meaning is shaped by culture. And it is clearly in part because of that social and cultural context that the impact on the individual is so enormous. Damaging, indeed, however, is a denial that disability does powerfully and negatively affect self-image and that a primary task for the disabled individual is to acknowledge and confront that reality.

I must define my own experience and, notwithstanding the importance of society and culture in shaping it, it remains mine. To say that there are no psychological consequences of disability (whatever their source or explanation) is to engage in denial of the most destructive kind. It was essential for me to admit to myself the impact of MS on my sense of who I was.

Contributing to the impact of MS on my sense of self-esteem and even identity were my strong fears about whether my intellectual capacity was, in fact, intact. This fear has not left me and returns with full force from time to time. The association between brain and intellect is quite properly very strong and, on a visceral level, it is hard for me not to assume that a damaged brain equals a damaged intellect, notwithstanding my lack of real evidence that my cognitive abilities have been damaged. There is some rational basis for this fear. Research has suggested that many persons with multiple sclerosis have some degree of undetected cognitive impairment.[4] This fear cuts to the very core of who I am and is not something I can be easy about. I cannot be reconciled to the thought that my mind might become impaired; the best I have been able to do is to accept that it is a possibility—however remote—and to be open to and learn to live with my fear. It is not something that is at the forefront of my consciousness all the time, but neither is it something that ever entirely goes away.

The continuing strength of that fear was brought home to me several years after my diagnosis when I took a day-long battery of very difficult tests in connection with an employment appli-

4. Charles M. Poser, "Multiple Sclerosis: A Critical Update," *Medical Clinics of North America: Symposium on Clinical Neurology* (July 1979): 740. See also Willem van den Burg et al., "Cognitive Impairment in Patients with Multiple Sclerosis and Mild Physical Disability," *Archives of Neurology* (May 1987): 494–501.

cation. I did very well on those tests and it was not until I heard the results that I realized how afraid I had been that my intellectual capacity had been damaged. This fear is heightened, of course, by the question of to what degree I would be aware of such damage or impairment or whether others would tell me. This raises interesting and age-old questions about consciousness and the limits of the self. In this connection, I recall being shown CT scan pictures of my brain. As the neurologist pointed out the areas of damage—the plaques caused by MS—I marveled at the notion of contemplating with my brain, my damaged brain.

The knowledge that my brain was damaged—the very center of my being—affected my entire image of myself and my integrity as a person. I felt less than whole and this was reflected by my hesitant behavior in all situations. I had always been an extremely competent person and yet I was feeling incompetent in situations that should have been second nature to me. It is difficult to convey the strength of these feelings; they can hardly be overstated. My whole notion of who I was was threatened and it was only very slowly that my feeling of disability began to be limited to the ways in which I was, objectively, disabled.

It is important to realize that one may have a very real sense of disability even when that disability is minimal and generally invisible to others. My disability *was* minimal, limited to difficulty in walking on occasion, a less than optimally functioning arm, balance problems, and unpredictable, if occasionally severe, fatigue. At the best of times, this was entirely invisible to others; at the worst of times, it was very visible as I stumbled along. But even at the best of times, it was always obvious to me that my arm and leg were not the way they "should" be and that I was not the way I once had been. And this sense of disability with its accompanying feeling of no longer being in control flowed over into all areas of my life.

My image of myself was altered. I had not realized—had not thought about—the ways, for example, in which my physical presentation of myself affected my self-image. I was more aware of the fact that my sense of self was very much bound up with my intellectual ability. But I had no sensitivity to the ways in which alteration in my physical self would affect my intellectual and emotional life. My difficulty with walking and my experience in graduate school were for me two of the more significant experiences that forced me to come to terms with the impact of the disease on my sense of self and to realize that while my brain might be damaged, my personhood need not be, and, in fact, could be enhanced. For others, it may be other kinds of experiences that lead them to this realization. Regaining my confidence was a very slow and painful process. Recognizing that multiple sclerosis had not only attacked my brain but had attacked my entire being was the first step. The second step was acknowledging the ways in which the physical changes had irrevocably changed me and affected my sense of self. And the third step was differentiating the physical and the emotional aspects of the impact of the disease.

The second crucial aspect of the process of acceptance is very closely related to the first, those issues of self-esteem and self-image, and involves the notion of "giving up." By this I mean accepting the changes and limitations the disease has imposed— what has been lost. I, for example, no longer stride quickly and energetically along the street. That is not one of the biggest things one can be required to give up, by any means, but it was part of me and it no longer is. I reluctantly and finally gave up the notion of getting a graduate degree. I was forced to recognize that I did not have the energy to work full-time, commute, and go to school at night. Giving that up was difficult; academic work was important to me and a part of my life. I have had to rethink my goals and aspirations. I have been very lucky in this regard; I have not had to give up anything that is absolutely central to my notion of myself and my place in the world. What if I were a professional tennis player who could no longer play tennis? My idea of who I am has never been very closely related to what I do, but if what was lost was central to one's identity, the struggle to redefine, or perhaps even to re-find, one's self would be enormous. And there are many who have had to do just that.

I had one experience that taught me a great deal about giving up, about self-image, and about what is really important. When I started graduate school, I was taking ACTH injections. The most noticeable side effects were that I gained a lot of weight (I have always been slim) and my face not only became puffy but changed shape. The degree of the change in my appearance was such that one mórning when I looked in the mirror, I failed to recognize myself. I looked nothing like my internal vision of myself. I was forced to realize, through observing the reactions of those I did not know, how much I had always relied on my physical appearance both to convey information about me to others and to carry me through situations. I looked stupid and ugly and I was suddenly being treated as stupid and ugly. That realization was entirely new to me and rather a shock. How much I had taken for granted. But, in the context of this discussion, the importance of the experience (the changes were temporary) was that I realized I could give that up, not easily and not without grief, but my appearance was not essential to who I was. There was some freedom in that recognition. And, once I realized that my appearance was not ultimately essential to my sense of self, it became easier to accept the other physical changes I was experiencing.

The process of giving up also involves reordering priorities. For me, the process started with the realization, described above, that my entire sense of self was affected by the knowledge that I had multiple sclerosis. And I soon realized that I had to think carefully, once again, about who I really was, what were the truly important things, and what were those things that, on reflection, were not all that significant. Once that has been done, it becomes much easier to give up that which is lost. Contemplating the possibility that in five years or ten years I may not be able to walk places the fact that I now walk with difficulty in perspective. More broadly, it enabled me to recognize that who I am is not dependent on my physical self, although the intimate and intricate relationship between the two is in some measure what this whole process is about. Forcibly reminded of the fragility of life, I began to pay more attention to those parts of life I deem most important. I learned a great deal about what is integral and integrating to me and I stopped wasting energy— physical or emotional—on those things that really do not matter.

To sum up so far, the emotional impact of multiple sclerosis can be staggering. The feeling of damage can involve the innermost reaches of one's psyche and affect one's entire approach to life. For me, the process of adjustment required searching examination of who I was and what it was that made me who I am. I had to learn that certain things that had seemed to be integral to my sense of self could be given up—that, for example, even when I looked stupid and ugly, I was still who I had been. Accepting the fact of this disease was a far-reaching and comprehensive process, probably never to be fully completed.

Having a very bad time after a period of feeling very well is sometimes like a recapitulation, albeit much faster, of the whole adjustment process. The first bad day is all too often a shock; I have forgotten what it was like, not only the purely physical aspects but the whole constellation of feelings and reactions. I forget and I have to remember exactly what is involved in living with chronic disease and with disability. Acceptance is an evolving, continuing, and often repetitive process. And while each cycle, as it were, holds within it all that has gone before, it also incorporates new experience and understandings. Acceptance is not an event or a task that once achieved is completed. There is no sequential progression from diagnosis to acceptance. I find myself forgetting this—forgetting even the existence of the process itself.

Another area in which the fact of this disease forced me to come to terms with some new realities and confront some very basic emotional issues was in recognizing the impact of my experience on my primary relationships and, to a lesser degree, on all my relationships. As with my own emotional life, issues and conflicts that had been worked out and confronted with a large degree of success suddenly seemed to be alive once again. The fact of multiple sclerosis and its impact on me had a significant effect on my relationships with others in ways that I would not have dreamed possible and was certainly not prepared for.

Dependence once again became an issue for me. The conflict between independence and dependence (common to many women of my generation) had, I thought, long since been acknowledged and resolved. Yes, there was a part of me that longed to be protected and taken care of; but, no, that was not dominant and I would not allow it to interfere with or structure my relationships. Now, however, not only was I faced with the very real possibility of physical dependence, but suddenly a large part of me seemed to be asking to be taken care of— indirectly, to be sure, but nonetheless it was real and I did not like it. Yet, at the same time, my fear of dependence was keeping me from asking for help when it would have been legitimate. And while my fear of becoming very sick and dependent increased my need for a safe place, for certainty in my emotional life, I was expressing that fear and those needs indirectly and inappropriately.

I also realized that for the first time I was really afraid of being left alone and that this fear was subtly affecting my relationships. Not only did I find myself implicitly asking to be taken care of but I was going to extraordinary lengths on occasion to please others in ways that I found to be dishonest as well as manipulative. I discovered that I was afraid to express my anger and I was uneasy about others' anger. I had thought that anger—my own and others—was something I'd learned to accept and deal with honestly and openly. Suddenly I found that my anger frightened me and the anger of others terrified me. I realized that I was afraid that people would leave me if I was honest about my anger or if they were angry with me, and my fear was of being left alone with this disease and its possible implications.

I also had a great fear of somehow blackmailing those I was close to—of using the fact of the disease in an underhanded way to get what I wanted. I was second-guessing others—not trusting them either to see me clearly or to be responsible for themselves. These were all issues that I thought had been worked out successfully years earlier, but which suddenly, under the impact of my disease, rose to the fore again.

One result of the disease for which I was thoroughly unprepared was its direct and extraordinary effect on my relationship with Nick. We had a strong relationship and I thought that the impact of the disease would be absorbed easily and with no major adjustments and that, insofar as there were difficulties, they would be my difficulties. I was wrong. At the time of my diagnosis I was briefly hospitalized to begin the course of ACTH injections. A series of incidents occurred over the first few days after I left the hospital which alerted us to the fact that something was going on which involved not my reactions to the disease but his. An exceptionally good-humored and easygoing man, Nick was suddenly becoming very angry in situations that normally would have caused exasperation at most. And to my dismay, much of his anger seemed to be directed at me. The level of his anger, and its indiscriminate nature, was so out of proportion to events that it alarmed us both.

We very slowly began to understand that his anger was not so much with me as on my behalf and arose from his feeling of helplessness. He loved me, wanted to be able to make things OK for me, and had difficulty acknowledging that my MS was something he could neither fix nor alleviate. He was angry with himself for not being able to help me, angry with the world in a vague sort of way for allowing this to happen to me, and angry with me as well for, in some obscure way, betraying him, letting him down by getting sick. He felt very helpless and he reacted by striking out at whatever got in his way—including me. In *The Wings of the Dove*, Henry James speaks of this as "the woe of learning the torment of helplessness."[5] Before Nick could come to terms with the fact of MS in my life, and before we could incorporate it into our relationship, he had first to acknowledge his anger and, more important, his powerlessness to change what had or what might happen. He wanted to make everything OK for me and he couldn't. That is a hard lesson to learn. In retrospect, this all seems very clear to both of us; at the time, it was very difficult.

We were both helped, strangely enough, by my difficulty in continuing with the ACTH injections. I had been taught to do it in the hospital, it had been very easy for me, and I'd not given much thought to continuing the injections at home. It became apparent very quickly, however, that giving myself an injection with a nurse standing by and doing it alone were two entirely

5. Henry James, *The Wings of the Dove* (New York: Penguin Books, 1965), p. 262.

different things. I had an extraordinarily difficult time and as the days passed it got harder, not easier.

Nick's response to all of this could not have been better. He neither belittled my difficulty nor took it more seriously than need be. He did not try to do it for me. He understood, as did I, that it was important that I do it by and for myself. Instead, by his presence, and his calm assurance that I could indeed do what was necessary, he made it possible for me to find and use my own strength. He was supportive in the truest possible sense of that word.

Going through that together was good for both of us. And it was really through that process that he realized that no, he could not—nor should he—do for me what I needed to do for myself, nor could he make everything OK for me. When he accepted his essential helplessness, his anger disappeared. But he also realized that by his presence, by his trust and belief in me, he could help to make it possible for me to do what I needed to do. And I not only realized how necessary that trust and support was but learned something about seeking and asking for the right kind of help.

Soon after this, an incident occurred which, seen in retrospect, contains elements of many of the issues that were raised anew in our relationship by the fact of MS in our lives. It has become symbolic for us and a reminder of the kinds of difficulties that can occur. One afternoon in a parking garage I watched him back his car out and smash his fender on a concrete pillar. No damage was done to his car and we joked about his ineptness. The next afternoon, I backed my car into the same pillar and, unfortunately, did a fair amount of damage. My first reaction was to burst into tears and I started to telephone him to ask for help. I immediately bit my mental tongue, realizing not only that I needed no help, but that even if I had a problem, I was perfectly capable of taking care of it myself, and drove home.

By the time I got home I had realized the funny side of the story and called him at his office. My intention was to say, "You won't believe the stupid thing I just did, after watching you do it yesterday and isn't this funny?" He, however, jumped right in and started yelling at me—"What do you expect me to do? You always expect me to fix everything for you"—and hung up on me. I was enraged not only at his assumptions but that he would make assumptions at all. He soon called back and we realized exactly what we had done. He had assumed I was calling for help, thought I was being manipulative by covering a request for help with a joke, asking for help when I did not really need it, and was angry. He had not bothered to listen to what I was saying. I was forced to realize that he had some reason for these assumptions. I had been relying on him heavily in both appropriate and inappropriate ways. He wanted to help me and was forced to learn that in many ways he could not. I wanted help and had to learn that what I was really asking for—to be made whole, to be taken care of, for security, emotional and physical—was not available. It took a while for us to sort out the ways in which help was available and those in which it was not.

This story was paradigmatic for us. It illuminated some of the ways in which the new fact of my disease and its effect on me were clouding our relationship. Yes, I was dependent in some new ways but that need not spill over into all areas of the relationship. He and I had learned the hard way years earlier not to make assumptions about the other's intentions, to be honest and direct in communicating our feelings, and to trust the other to be responsible for his own feelings and needs. All of a sudden, it seemed that we had forgotten the very basis of our relationship—trust and honesty—and it took something silly like our bent fender incident to remind us of what we were doing.

I had to realize the ways in which I was imposing on this relationship and others the conflicts and struggles I was experiencing as a result of multiple sclerosis. I had to learn the ways in which my experience did affect relationships and the ways in which it need not. I had to recognize, for example, that my great need for certainty and security, while understandable and legitimate, could be seen for what it was and need not be allowed to muddy relationships. I had to come to terms with my fears, my need for security, and I had to do it by myself.

While the impact of the disease on me affected my closest relationships most strongly, I soon discovered that it had an impact on all my relationships in one way or another. Almost without thinking, I immediately told all my relatives and friends that I had multiple sclerosis. My thinking, such as it was, was that it was a major event in my life and insofar as it affected me, it would affect my relationships. I think I also thought that telling people would get it out of the way and, in some fashion, divest it of some of its importance to me. I am not sorry I did it that way—I received a lot of support and reassurance that might not otherwise have been available. I discovered that almost everyone I talked to knew someone with multiple sclerosis and I learned a great deal and was reassured by the stories I heard. There is also a sense in which telling people and dealing with their reactions forced me to confront the disease more quickly than I might otherwise have done.

I made mistakes, one of which haunts me to this day because it is such a stark example of exactly what I do not want to do or become. Soon after my diagnosis, when I was feeling exceedingly unattractive and miserable from the side effects of ACTH, I met an old friend in the supermarket. I had not seen her for several years and she routinely asked how I was. I blurted out that I was miserable, thank you, and that I had multiple sclerosis. Her face fell, she muttered something, and walked away. I realized that I had done something totally unnecessary and self indulgent. I could just as easily have responded, "Fine, thank you." The question was routine, so, too, could have been my answer. Telling her I had MS was purely gratuitous. From time to time, I have told others whom, on reflection, there was no need to tell. I think I would be a little more selective and a little more careful about timing were I able to do it again.

However, I was totally unprepared for the range of reactions I received or their force. It seemed at times as though it took more emotional energy and wisdom to deal with my friends' reactions than it was taking to accept the disease myself. And it had never occurred to me that telling someone about the disease could cause difficulties for them in our relationship. Although, in retrospect, I suppose I might have been more sensitive, this is one of those issues that no one sees as important enough to mention at the outset but which is difficult to foresee and is important.

The day I learned the diagnosis, I spent the evening with two of my closest friends. I was in shock and totally unable to focus on, much less discuss, anything else, and told them what had happened as I walked in the door. Their reaction was to fail to acknowledge what I said. They hardly said a word, but it was very clear that they would not only not discuss it, they did not want me to talk about it. They simply and totally ignored what I was saying. These were sensitive, caring people who had been good friends of mine for years. I felt very let down, very alone, and I was not able that night to understand their reaction. It only became clear to me later that they were angry and frightened themselves and had no idea how to respond to my (not so implicit) needs that night.

I encountered varying reactions in the next few weeks from close friends and relatives whom I told of my disease. Responses ranged from denial, generally taking the form of a refusal to talk with me about it or even to listen to me, to anger. The anger astounded me, as it seemed to be directed at me. Other reactions I encountered included: "Yes, so what"; something I called "the end-of-the-world" reaction; and even disappointment—"But you don't look sick."

One angry reaction came from a very close friend and, at first, I perceived only the fact of his anger and that it seemed to be directed at me. I finally realized that what he was saying was, in essence, "How could you do this to me?" He had relied on me always to be there when he needed me, and to be strong, and he now felt, apparently, that I was unreliable. He felt abandoned and was angry about it. He also, like Nick, was angry that something had happened to me and he could do nothing about it. It took me a while to realize this, though, and my first reaction was to feel very hurt. I finally asked him whether, in fact, he was angry with me and he admitted that he was. We talked about it at some length. Once he realized that I remained who I had been, and acknowledged his anger to himself, we were able to be good friends again. But reaching that point took a lot of time and energy.

The "yes, so what?" reaction has always fascinated me. It usually takes the form of a recital of that person's own symptoms and medical history—an "everything you've got, I've got more of" response. I have often wondered whether it is intended as a form of comfort or whether it is another reflection of fear, of not wanting to know that such things can happen. On the other hand, there are those who respond as though disaster is imminent and seem to want me to act very sick. No matter what I say or do, they relate to me as though I were sick. One friend continues to urge me to retire because of disability when it should be perfectly obvious that I am capable of working.

There have been some people whose response to learning that I have multiple sclerosis is complete aversion. A good example of this was the casual acquaintance I chatted with for a couple of hours in a social setting. There came a time in the conversation when the fact of my MS seemed relevant and I referred to it. He said, "Why didn't you tell me that before?" and immediately walked away. Some of this aversion seems attributable to a fear of contagion. This is difficult to pin down, of course, primarily because those who react in this way do abruptly leave.

There were people who responded perfectly. They let me talk about it when I needed to, let me voice my fear without either belittling it or being themselves afraid of my fear. They were sorry this had happened to me and said so and they conveyed real acceptance and gave me real support. They treated me no differently than they ever had. Thinking back, these were people who were both very aware and very accepting of who they themselves were.

These varying responses were my introduction to the whole notion of what it means to be sick or, more accurately, to be perceived as sick, in this culture and of how difficult it can be to retain a feeling of integrity in the face of these responses. There is ambiguity in a chronic disease such as MS—one is sick but not sick; one is sick at some times and healthy at others; and one's physical appearance is not necessarily reflective of either state. My belief that the diagnosis, that discrete and clarifying event, would clear up all the confusion in my world of relationships began to be confounded.

In many of these encounters I felt as though people were reacting more to the fact of the disease than to me and that at those times, a screen had been erected between me and the world. I was not seen then as a person with a disease; the disease alone was seen and people responded to it in what I began to see as fairly predictable ways.

I was reminded very quickly that people fear reminders of their own vulnerability and, ultimately, of their mortality. And because most people know very little about multiple sclerosis, they tend to assume that the outcome will be immediately devastating. Many women of my age seemed to react by thinking, if this can happen to you, it can happen to me, and since I don't want to acknowledge that, I will just deny that it has happened to you. Many people also firmly believe that this (MS or whatever) happens only to someone else, a defense that is only effective if enough distance and separation is maintained.

All this occurred at a time when I was very needy and stunned. But I found myself being forced to listen carefully and try to understand what was behind some of these reactions. It was undoubtedly very good for me to be forced to think of something other than myself. And there was a lot of comic relief; many of these encounters were very funny. Trying to understand what was going on was very useful to me in my understanding of my own reactions to the disease. At the time, however, it was very trying and required a lot of emotional energy I didn't have. And it had simply not occurred to me that this was part of what the disease would involve. I had had the notion that I would tell friends and they would be supportive and caring and that would be that. Most of my friends ultimately were just that, but it was not a simple process.

Throughout this time, I was reminded of how rare and wonderful it is to be unconditionally loved and accepted. There were many times during this process when I was not particularly lovable and yet I was loved and accepted by those closest to me. I learned especially to value those few who openly conveyed this unconditional acceptance and love and who gave me an enormous amount of support without in any way trying to do for me what I had to do for myself. Those were the people who enabled me to find and use my own strength.

After learning that I had multiple sclerosis, I was faced with a period of significant change and adjustment. The medical professionals I came in contact with, for whom I have great respect, not only gave me no warning of what could be involved, but consistently implied that no significant adjustment was necessary. This implication, in itself, made the process more difficult because I wondered whether I was overreacting. In retrospect, I don't think that I was and I think that the process I went through in coming to terms with the knowledge of the disease is, in general terms, very common. There is a lack of information about this process and I believe it is important that such information be available to newly diagnosed persons.

The immediate process of adjustment to multiple sclerosis required identifying those areas of my life that were changed by the fact of the disease and then adjusting to those changes. It required recognition of the ways in which I was changed and the ways in which the disease and my reactions to it affected my relationships. It required a new level of clarity and honesty as I looked at who I was and how my whole being was affected. I was forced to look very closely at what I was doing as I tried to fully accept the implications of having multiple sclerosis. Multiple sclerosis is not the primary fact of my life—significant, yes, but I am not and I refuse to be an "MS person." It took a lot of time and effort, however, before I truly came to terms with the implications of the disease.

By identifying the areas in which the disease did make a difference, I was able to gain some clarity about the areas of my life where it is not—and need not be—a factor. It is important to keep the fact of the disease and its accompanying constellation of feelings from affecting those parts of life and living where it need not be an intrusive factor. But before I could do that, it was necessary to fully accept the ways in which it did change my life.

Multiple sclerosis, though not usually a fatal disease, does bring one face to face with the unavoidable but unacceptable knowledge of one's mortality and fragility. Becoming reconciled to the unacceptable is a slow and difficult process and requires new levels of self-knowledge. Throughout this process (and I don't mean to suggest it is complete—I imagine it is lifelong), I was beset by feelings of uncertainty as to whether my emotional responses were "normal." As I stumbled through these changes and discoveries, it would have been not only reassuring but positively helpful to know that my reactions were to be expected. There would have been a great deal of support in the recognition that what I was experiencing was natural and necessary. The process, I think, could have been shortened.

After I had achieved some degree of equilibrium and had begun to integrate the fact of MS into my life, I began to think more about some of the larger issues and questions raised by disease and disability in contemporary American life. The issues I mentioned earlier became pressing ones for me as I slowly realized that acceptance and adjustment on this personal level was not enough to live with any ease with chronic illness.

# Beyond the Self: The Cultural Frame

*. . . the intuition of the human situation itself,
more powerfully apprehended in the erection of a cultural bridge
than it might otherwise be.*
BRADD SHORE

Several years passed after my diagnosis before I realized how significantly my experience was being shaped by my culture. The crystallizing event in that realization was a month spent in the Middle East. It took perhaps the combination of being in another, foreign culture and being away from my own to make clear to me the impact of culture on my experience. It was only through stepping away and coming back that I saw myself in this larger context.

I had, until this time, tended to think about what was happening to me in purely individual terms, not as unique to me, of course, but as bounded by me and my social world—me and my disease, a definable unit, something apart from the realm of culture. I had been aware of some of the social consequences, particularly the impact on those I was close to, but I had not thought clearly about the ways in which their reactions and responses as well as my own were culturally shaped or socially demanded. I think perhaps it was necessary first to identify and begin to come to terms with the more personal and immediate issues. After I returned from the Middle East, my intuitive feelings about the ways in which others had viewed and had written about their experience with MS began to achieve some clarity and form.

Once I began to think about my experience in its cultural frame, I tried in some ways to keep it to myself, to retain its individual character. Increasingly, however, the relationship between my everyday life and the set of generally shared ideas, values, and symbols that constitutes my culture (for want of a better word) became apparent. It may seem that this should have been obvious but in this context it was not—at least to me. As this happened, I began to be aware of the conflicts between my life with a chronic disease and the values of the society in which I lived.

When I was in Egypt, walking with difficulty and using a cane, strangers and passersby asked me directly, "What is wrong with you? Why do you limp? Why are you sitting there? Why are you using a cane?" Walking in a Cairo street, an old woman came up to me, put her arm on mine, pointed to the cane, and patted my hand. I was struck by this; in the United States people don't ask questions of that nature or respond openly to disability. Instead they stare at or ignore me. The open acceptance I experienced in Egypt contrasted starkly with the equally open turning away I have come to expect in this country.

A brief example: one evening, riding on the commuter bus, surrounded by people I saw every day and who always smiled and chatted, I was unable to stand up. I eventually struggled out of my seat and stumbled to the door. Not one of these friendly people offered a hand; without exception, they averted their eyes and pretended not to notice my difficulty. Disease or disability is not something we openly acknowledge, but something we turn away from (this turning away is, of course, a form of acknowledgment).

My time in Egypt had a dramatic effect on me, although I only realized its impact after I had come home. I had felt so free and easy there. I had been just who I was, limped and stumbled about, and had *no* feelings about it. People reacted to me with care and consideration but so quietly, so matter-of-factly, that I wasn't aware of these differences until I came home. In Israel, in many ways a very Western society, I was completely ignored. No one modified their normal pushing and shoving behavior for me—everyone in Israel wants to be first in line—and I was knocked about quite often. That kind of being ignored is very different from what happens here, however, because it does not seem to be reflective of aversion. It is a not-seeing, not a seeing followed by a turning away.

What was important to me about being in the Middle East was the way in which it illuminated for me both the usual manner in which I am responded to here and the way I feel about it—my feelings had always been there, but I hadn't verbalized them even to myself and I hadn't thought very clearly about exactly what is being reflected by people's behavior. Moreover, I had not thought at all about these responses and my reactions to them in the context of my own acceptance and adjustment to chronic disease.

Another commuter bus example: I have trouble walking on a moving bus and tend to lurch around and bounce off people and seats and, of course, like everything else with MS, my difficulty varies from day to day. Over a period of several weeks I had engaged in normal bus conversation—about the weather, what we were reading—with a man who always took a seat near the rear of the bus, as I did. We had become increasingly friendly. One afternoon, when my difficulty moving was extreme, I fell getting off and he looked away. After that day that man, who had been very friendly, changed his seat and never even acknowledged a hello from me. I felt and still feel set apart, judged.

I've thought sometimes that people, in such situations, think I am drunk. I find myself trying very hard to walk straight, not to stumble or fall. I don't like being reacted to in that way and I like even less my response, my feelings of inadequacy, of being less than OK. Of course, there is always the possibility that nothing is happening in such a situation at all except someone deciding, for whatever reason, that they no longer want to be friendly, and that I, being always aware of the ways in which I am not "normal," filter all experience through that awareness. But I think not. I think that man, and many others, do react to disability with aversion.

I had a very strong urge in that particular situation to confront that man and ask him directly why he had ceased to speak to me. I didn't do that, both out of fear (he might, after all, have said, "Hey, lady—I just don't like you") and out of a sense of weariness; I didn't at the time think it was worth it and, after all, one cannot go around confronting everyone who responds with avoidance.

Another very common reaction is that of embarrassment. But I think embarrassment, like anger, is one of those emotions that is not in and of itself very meaningful. One is embarrassed because one is feeling something else. The range of feelings that are covered by embarrassment include fear, helplessness, powerlessness, distaste, pity; they are all subsumed by aversion. One may look away because one feels helpless but, whatever the reason, one is looking away.

Obscene—illness, disability, disease are seen as obscene. A friend suggested that the meaning of "obscene" is "to turn away from;" etymologically that is incorrect but intuitively it is right on the mark. "Obscene" means not only "repulsive" but "abhorrent to morality or virtue." What exactly was going on when a co-worker asked, "What happened to your leg?" and I (feeling weary of being asked and a bit bitchy) responded, "Nothing is wrong with my leg; I have multiple sclerosis." The response, and there is nothing uncommon about it, was "Sorry I asked" as he walked away. I can understand that response. Nevertheless, I felt rejected. I felt exactly as though I, in some fashion, affronted him; as though I was a reproach; as though I was, most of all, something that he did not wish to see or acknowledge.

And why is that? I have come to think it is at least partly because disease does not fit in the American world view and, in fact, conflicts so sharply as to create a situation in which comfort requires that it not be seen. Disease is, in fact, an affront. For to acknowledge it would require acknowledging that our most closely held values are, at their root, disconsonant with reality. "Cognitive dissonance" is the term psychologists use to describe such a situation. The common response is to ignore the potential conflict—to deny it. Disease is abhorrent to morality and virtue in the sense that it is ultimately beyond our control, and to acknowledge that would call into question our most central notions about life and nature. We turn away from disease because it is an affront to the way things should be.

I turn away, too. I am not immune. The only difference is that when I react that way, I am only too painfully aware of my reaction and its implications and try very hard to check it. I feel both my own instinct to turn away and the feelings in me when I am turned away from. And I stand there and ask myself why, and feel even more helpless because if I, who am turned away from, turn away from someone else, where is there an answer? I know that part of my reaction involves a not wanting to know and part of it is a helplessness, a not knowing what to do. And even though I know what it is I would like in the same situation, I don't (nor can I) know what a particular person in a given situation would like. I am sure that uncertainty contributes to what I experience as aversion.

I said earlier that help was abundantly available to me; that may seem to conflict with what I am saying here. I don't think there is a conflict. Help is offered by close friends and family when it is asked for and even when it is not. On the day-to-day, ordinary falling-on-the-bus level, however, help is not offered. In either of the two situations I recounted, I imagine that if, but only if, I had directly asked for help it would have been forthcoming. But help has to be asked for; it is not offered silently or casually in this culture. Rarely does anyone reach out a hand to steady someone unasked.

The presence or absence of large numbers of people seems to make a big difference. I once fainted and fell getting off a train in Grand Central Station—there were hundreds of people around—and I lay there, being carefully stepped over, until I managed some minutes later to get to my feet. In contrast, at those times when I have fallen in the presence of one or two people, generally, though not always, they have helped me. I think this difference is important (and of course, it also has to do with issues of individual and group psychology). It points up not only the distinction between individual actions and the generally held, generally shared thrust of the culture, but also the power of culture and society to shape and direct individual experience. In a group situation, the values of the group, as group, seem to prevail. Another factor that seems to be involved in determining whether I am offered help in day-to-day situations is whether or not I am carrying a cane. Help is more often offered when I am. A cane seems to act as a status marker, to confer legitimacy. It defines its bearer as someone who is not quite "normal."

I think here, however, of the many times I have offered help to a blind person crossing a street and been brusquely rejected—

"I can manage by myself"—or the acquaintance in a wheelchair who deeply resents anyone offering to help her. These people fiercely guard their independence. Does the fact that I am so rarely offered help reflect, in part, a generalized perception by others that I do not want it and would, in fact, reject it? In my generation, we were taught as Boy and Girl Scouts to offer that kind of help, the one good deed a day. My recollection, though, is that this help was to be directed primarily to the elderly. And, of course, there is always the "but you look so good" element at play in people's reactions to me. I usually do look well even when I am struggling to walk.

Apart from group dynamics, there are more fundamental reasons for these responses, which, I believe, are deeply rooted in the basic values and assumptions of this culture. An explanation of my difficulty in asking for help is also to be found in these basic values. I am not an expert on Middle Eastern culture and my time there was brief. But I suspect that one of the central factors underlying the differences I perceived is that in Egypt life rests on a very fatalistic approach; whatever will happen will happen: *Insh'allah*, God willing. Here, in contrast, the prevailing assumption is that an individual can determine what will happen. Fatalism versus free will, together with the strong emphasis on individual autonomy in American culture, are, I think, at the root of the differences I felt.

The other aspect of the freedom I felt in Egypt has to do with the fact that I was a foreigner, an outsider, there. I was not expected to know the rules of that culture or to be competent within it. And beyond that, there is a sense in which for me, my self was less at stake; the Egyptians did not know the usual criteria for evaluating it and, therefore, accepted me as I was. I was given an exemption, so to speak, from Egyptian rules and was not judged by my own rules either. V. S. Naipaul, an Indian, described this feeling perfectly when he spoke of visiting an island with no Indian population and therefore, "for me, no personal complication . . . I was just a stranger. . . . Judgments could be as simple as that there."[1] The parallel is imperfect

1. V. S. Naipaul, "The Enigma of Arrival," *The New Yorker*, 11 August 1986, p. 54.

but that lack of personal complication, that leaving behind the usual framework of life and self, was what allowed me to begin to see the complexities and conflicts inherent in my life at home.

I remember one day shortly after my return from the Middle East having to take both a subway and a bus to get home. I usually do not use the subway and I wasn't sure where I was going and felt very uncertain. I remember saying to myself, "Hey, I just traveled all over Egypt and felt perfectly competent—in an unknown country where I couldn't even read the signs. And yet, here I am in my own city feeling totally at sea." Part of that was, of course, that in Egypt I wasn't supposed to be competent, while here competence is expected. There is also the feeling in Egypt, which I found very catching and appealing, that if incompetence triumphs, so what? In this country there is much less tolerance for incompetence or inefficiency. At those times when I am particularly shaky and find it difficult to get around, I feel very vulnerable to that lack of tolerance.

The more important part of this, and the more curious for me, is that I, my self, my personhood, do seem to be at stake here. And it occurred to me to wonder just why that is so. What was it about having MS that had changed me? I never felt completely in tune with mainstream American culture or values. My values were different and I was always something of an outsider. But I had never felt judged or particularly in conflict with my culture or vulnerable to its assessments. Or perhaps, to be more accurate, I had not cared very much if I was out of tune with my culture. It was only when I came back from the Middle East that I began to feel the full force of these conflicts, to realize that I did feel my self was in some measure at stake. Suddenly, it did seem to matter when, for example, I am judged to be incompetent even in so small a thing as being lost on the subway.

I have great difficulty functioning in very warm weather and am apt to become confused and disoriented in extreme heat. And, of course, when that happens, I may well not be aware that I am in fact confused. One hot July day, I got off my bus as usual to transfer to another (do all my adventures take place on buses?). There were six or seven buses waiting and, for whatever reason—it was hot, I was tired—I did not find the bus I should have boarded. I suddenly became aware that everyone else had boarded a bus, the transfer area was empty, and I was wandering from bus to bus. Everyone was waiting for me. None of this had registered. I immediately climbed aboard the closest bus and then realized it was the one I had been on before. People were looking at me as though I were crazy. I felt judged and a failure, incompetent.

The point of this story is twofold. First, had it happened in Egypt, I would not have been held to the same level of expectation by others because I was an outsider. A bus that leaves on time, that runs at all, is an accomplishment in Egypt. Efficiency is surely not expected, and therefore if I had caused a delay, it would have not mattered at all to anyone. Second, I was quite clearly seen as incompetent by my fellow commuters in that situation, even as something of a public nuisance because I had delayed all the buses. But why did it matter so much to me? I began to realize that my new sense of vulnerability and the feeling that I was being held up against a set of values and feeling incongruent with them, in both big and small ways, arose in large measure out of my awareness and fear of my potential dependency. It was the clarity I found in Egypt, suddenly removed from the constraints and the usual framework of living, that led me to see these issues so starkly.

After I returned home, I began to think about what it means to be disabled in America. What are the prevailing values and underlying assumptions of this culture and how do they affect my daily life? My experience is shaped and, in some measure, controlled by living within the frame of these assumptions and it suddenly seemed very important to examine them more closely.

Several common assumptions come to mind, all rooted in the American ethic of self-determination: we are what we do; we have self-responsibility and autonomy; we can control our life and experience—outcomes are controllable. Illness and disease are seen as punishment; the idea exists that failure implies a defect in character and will.

What are the primary values of American culture on which these assumptions are based? Values are notoriously hard to define or measure, in part because a group's dominant values may conflict with how it lives on a daily basis. What we like to or need to think we are may not bear much relation to what we are in fact. Important symbols may encapsulate values that are not operative in daily life but that are crucially important in how we think about ourselves. Moreover, the dominant values of a group will be variously represented among individuals; there may be wide variations in beliefs, practices, expressed values. "Values" may well be the wrong word to use here, but I think it is as useful as any other concept in thinking about the impact of culture on individual experience. Values reflect common understandings and shared assumptions about the world and the nature of reality within which and through which experience is filtered.

There are four primary values that I have come to see as paramount and all-encompassing in shaping and coloring the experience of being ill in America. I think these values are basic to and underlie the working assumptions of this culture. The first, and probably the most important, is the notion that humans both do and should control nature and that control, on all levels, is always a desired outcome. The high value given to control is central to the common understanding of illness and disability in America. Second, and akin to the value given to control, is the centrality of the idea of independence and self-sufficiency. Independence is highly valued in this culture. It is both desired and seen as an achievable outcome. It is more important in terms of how we think about ourselves and in how we react to others than in the realities of our lives. Nevertheless, as one of the central ideas in this culture, the perceived autonomy of the individual is key. The third basic value is to be found in the dominance given to the future over both the present and the past. Future implies change, which in and of itself is highly valued. Change is perceived both as always possible and as a consistently desired outcome. Tomorrow will always be bigger and better. The fourth important value is activity. Doing is highly valued in American culture and doing, as opposed to being, is a primary response to almost anything.

These values and the assumptions that flow from them about the nature of reality provide a useful framework against which to think about what it means to be sick or disabled in this culture as well as about how disease is viewed. I also think that less important but inextricably entwined with these values and a significant element in what it means to be ill in this culture is a subsurface and covert belief that disease both reflects and results from an inherent imperfection or flaw in human nature.

Disease and disability do not fit easily within the American value system. There is almost total conflict. As I considered my experience in the light of these values, I began to see some faint glimmers of light illuminating the roots of the conflicts I felt. Suddenly one's experience—who it is that I am today—is radically at odds with governing assumptions about reality and life. Part of the difficulty in coming to terms with that break, that discontinuity, is that precisely because I am a part of this society, have been shaped by its values, and have grown up in a world that is bounded by these assumptions, the potential for conflict is so strong. The more I am congruent with my culture and have internalized its dominant thrust, the more conflict there will be when suddenly my experience is at odds with it. The paradox, of course, is that the greater the conflict, the less acknowledgment of it there may be and the stronger the need to overcome or at least to appear to overcome it.

It is at the intersection of this conflict—between American values and disease—that denial arises. In a situation where realities conflict, either one of them must be changed or disregarded or there must be an accommodation and adjustment to the fact of the conflict. In this context, the culture cannot be changed, nor can the fact that one has a disease. Denial is an easier response than its alternative, acceptance. Over time, however, denial is more stressful, requires more energy to maintain, and is ultimately self-defeating. My initial and primarily intuitive understanding of why hope, arising out of or leading to denial, was such a common response to MS in the books I read began to make sense as I considered this conflict between the reality of chronic disease and the primary values of American society.

One of the first things that a chronic disease such as MS forces one to realize is that nature is not controllable. Yet the belief that nature is, and should be, controllable by humankind is absolutely central to this culture. I have no control over the disease activity in my brain. In and of itself, this is hard enough to accept, but acceptance does come. That acceptance is infinitely harder to achieve, however, when the culture continually—in both small and big ways—tells me that I should be in control, that control is possible, and that accepting or believing that I am not in control is a giving up, a moral failure, and an affirmation of the fact that my nature is flawed.

The conflict between chronic disease and the value given to the future in this culture is fairly straightforward. For me, today is important. I have no way of knowing what will happen to me; the fact that I am walking today is of overriding importance to me. Change would certainly be nice, but if I rely on the possibility of change, the hope of improvement, then I fail to live fully today. Again, this society—in all its voices, books, the media, friends, family, even leftover bits of me—constantly tells me not to give up hope of change and moreover, would have me make that hope a centerpiece of my life. Certainly I hope that a cure for MS will be found but I cannot live in that hope. Given the realities of this disease, chances are very good that the future may not be better; it may not be worse but it is not likely to be better. Yet a very common response to disease in this culture is talk of overcoming it or of conquering it. The stories are legion about people who have "won the battle" against disease. With a chronic disease such as MS, this is not a very helpful approach.

The other aspect of this emphasis on the future that I find to be in conflict with my experience and my expectations is the notion that the future will take care of itself; again, the implication is that the future will be better than the present. My view of the future is radically different now than it was before I knew I had MS. The future has constricted and the range of possibility seems narrower. Of course, I am also rapidly becoming middle-aged and, with age, the future does become less open-ended. This is true for everyone but is much more acute with chronic disease. I am more concerned with providing for the possibilities of the future than with hope of change and improvement.

The possibility, however remote, that I might become more

disabled led me to take a large salary cut to get into the federal civil service because I felt it provided the greatest degree of employment security available for the disabled. Others urge me to take bigger career risks in the hope that all will be well and the future will take care of itself. I do not feel that I can do that. There is an element of contradiction here because while I feel I must be cognizant of the worst that might happen and prepare for that, I also feel enormous pressure to live for today, to enjoy life to its fullest while I can. The conflict for me becomes this: if I have some money, do I use it to go to Egypt while I am still able to walk or do I save it for the day when I might be unable to work? In either event, the cultural message that the future will be an improvement over the present is totally at odds with my understanding of reality.

It is certainly true that change is often feared. Nevertheless, even then there remains an underlying belief in and assumption of progress. Things change, they progress; and whether change is welcomed or not, this is one of the most important operating assumptions of this society—of most of the Western world, for that matter. Radiating out from the extraordinary impact of Darwin's work on evolutionary processes into all areas of culture, this belief has permeated our thinking. Change, and in the form of progress, is seen as inevitable. Those with chronic disease live, on whatever level and whether perceived or not, in opposition to this assumption. The progression of disease will not be in a positive direction for the individual.

An outgrowth of this preoccupation with the future is the high value American society gives to time, per se. Time is valuable, time is money. And I can be very slow and get in people's way. On a train in Egypt, my friend and I asked the waiter what time dinner would be served. "*Insh'allah,*" he replied. "OK," we said, "that's fine, we'll be in the club car." "No, no, no," he said. "You'll miss dinner." He had already shown his grave disapproval of two women sitting in the club car for any reason, much less our expressed reason—to have a drink. "We'll stay," we said, "if dinner is soon." "Oh," he said, "Soon? Dinner will be . . . *Insh'allah.*" So we persisted, and every twenty minutes or so one of us would go to our car to check on dinner. The waiter each time said, "Come back, come back." We'd ask if dinner was ready and he, stretched out and smoking a cigarette in the kitchenette, would smile and say, "*Insh'allah.*" I think we had dinner about three hours later. I loved every moment of Egypt. Time as time has no value there.

The emphasis on doing in this culture is equally in conflict with the experience of a chronic disease such as MS and is closely related to the high value placed on the future. Activity is prized and judgments are based on what one does. The question most often asked at a cocktail party is, "What do you do?" Similarly, "Let's do something about it" or "What are you doing about it?" are stock phrases in this culture. They reflect an understanding about the nature of reality that is widespread. Accepting that there is nothing that can be done and refusing to engage in futile attempts to change what is put one in an uncomfortable position. I hear constantly that acceptance is passive and weak; to rage and fight would be much more acceptable. Doing anything is far more acceptable than doing nothing.

These three primary values—that men and women control nature, that the future will be better, and that activity is the preferred response—are all related. Activity, doing something about it, rests on the understanding that nature can be controlled, something can always be done, and tomorrow will be better than today. Highlighting the future implies the possibility and efficacy of action.

Finally, living with chronic disease makes it impossible to continue to believe that individual autonomy and independence are possible, even if one considers them desirable. Dependence is an all too real and potential outcome. I am not autonomous now; I am dependent on my friends in many ways. Although I value my independence and try to maintain it, I also try to remember that independence, in and of itself, cannot be a central issue for me. I think this is made much more difficult by the fact that dependence carries with it very negative overtones and, indeed, has a negative meaning for me too. Because of this, I tend to go to great lengths to avoid the appearance of dependence and, therefore, make my life more difficult and complicated than it need be. Both the full implications of this issue and its complexity continue to become apparent to me.

The notion that human nature is basically flawed is, I think, connected to the subsurface but strong belief in American culture that disease is a manifestation of a break in the proper scheme of things and, moreover, is a form of punishment. A common response in the face of illness or misfortune is, "What have I done to deserve this?" We do seem to think that there must be a reason for misfortune and that this reason rests at the level of moral cause and effect. If I accept, then, that I have a chronic disease, it seems that I accept the imperfection of my nature. In this context, multiple sclerosis is quite neutral when compared with AIDS, which is overtly seen as a moral outcome and a punishment, or with cancer, which also carries with it some of these connotations. There is a very strong undercurrent to the effect that one gets exactly what one deserves.

On the surface, however, we think of ourselves as viewing disease scientifically, in physical cause-and-effect terms, and it is important to us that we do think this way. We believe that cures for all disease are available; it is only a question of when, and the when ultimately rests on the degree of will and resources we devote to the task. The extraordinary results of modern science and technology support this. A cure for cancer, a vaccine against AIDS, will be found if only we work hard enough. We overtly treat disease as a scientific problem to be solved. We assert that our response to disease is untainted by moral notions of cause and effect and is primarily rational.

We do think that there is no real distinction between our scientific and folk notions of illness and disease. Although we profess to view disease entirely in scientific terms, we actually (if covertly) view it also in moral terms. Disease is both a derangement of the proper relationship of humans to nature—of humankind subjugating nature to its will—and a reflection of that unimproved nature.

It is precisely because disease is covertly viewed as a moral outcome that it is dealt with as a purely physical issue. If we were to acknowledge to ourselves and to each other that we see disease in other than scientific terms, a great many of the things we hold central would be seen as standing on very fragile ground. Our world view, much of what it is most important to us to affirm, would be shaken. I think that there is an enormous discrepancy between how we really think and feel about these things and how we tell ourselves we feel, how we profess to feel. Under the impact of something as personally overwhelming as the knowledge of chronic disease or disability these conflicts become apparent.

There is a clear relationship between the view of disease as a moral issue and religion. Certainly, Judeo-Christian thought has had a significant influence on the development of American culture and values and does continue on some level to be important. And I think it clear that the mainstream religions in this country not only support the conflicts I feel but have added to them. While the theological basis of religion may be viewed as less influential today, the impact of Christianity lies in the ways in which it has contributed to shaping American values and is woven into the entire cultural system. Contemporary American religions do continue to support and legitimate what it is that people want to do and to give an underpinning and a rationale to their fears (for example, the fundamentalist response to AIDS). Religions are constantly re-created in forms that more closely meet the needs of their adherents.

Religion both keeps alive and supports the notion that disease is a moral issue. There is a not very subtle thread in Christianity, which I think has long been entrenched in the culture as a whole, to the effect that disease and suffering are deserved. They are also viewed as good in and of themselves in that they promote a desired moral outcome. Witness Pope John Paul II speaking at Lourdes to an audience of people in wheelchairs and on stretchers, as he urged them to accept their infirmities as a "special mission" and "interior liberation" that lets them lose themselves in divine love "for the sake of humanity."[2]

A relative of mine, on hearing that I had MS, referred me to Romans 5:3, where St. Paul writes that suffering produces endurance, endurance promotes character, and character, in turn, produces hope. The implication, hard to ignore, was twofold. First, my character needed improving, and I don't think it is far-

2. Quoted in Henry Kamm, "Pope at Lourdes, Seeks to Console the Suffering," *New York Times*, 16 August 1983, p. 3.

fetched to see an element of punishment here. After all, were I not in need of improvement, did I not lack character, or were it not deficient, I would not be in need of suffering ultimately to improve it. Second, hope is essential. And, as always, hope, of change or of improvement, seems to be the ultimate goal. Hope is an end in itself.

The notion that disease indicates a flawed relationship with God and is to be accepted as a consequence thereof is also common. If one's nature is flawed, then disease is a reflection of that. But religion also lets everyone off the hook. For the sick or disabled, there is the hope of future redemption and future change, a hope strongly supported by the cultural emphasis on the future. Acceptance is not necessary. Moreover, because hope is the goal and acceptance makes hope unnecessary, acceptance is somehow wrong. The Christian emphasis on hope is clearly related to belief in eternal life; one might even see this as the American emphasis on the future carried to its ultimate degree. In this regard, at least, the two systems fit together very nicely. Eternal life certainly is an important underpinning of hope and, if death is overcome, then it is less important to deal with life as it is.

For society at large, there is both the idea that illness is deserved and the God's-will theory. And if, indeed, disease reflects God's will and is deserved, then why should humans not accept it—as long as it happens to someone else. But the message is very mixed: accept and don't accept. If you are sick, then presumably there is a metaphysical reason for it and that may well be God's will and a reflection of his judgment; on the other hand, hope is the ultimate goal. A reliance on hope obviates the need for any real acceptance. This is very confused and I think the confusion is in the culture. It is another example of a situation in which real clarity would do damage to our basic understanding of ourselves and would force us to question the underpinnings of our belief system. And so we avoid clarity and accept confusion.

The perpetual quest for meaning, which can be so destructive of adjustment to chronic disease or illness of any kind, also arises out of this complex of beliefs. One commonly hears why?—why did this baby die? why is this young woman dying of cancer? People seem to need to find an overarching meaning in these things and construct elaborate edifices to provide it and to protect them from the harshness of reality—Peter Berger's notion of religion as a sacred canopy. For believers, meaning is too easily found in the notion (however unacknowledged and hidden) that disease is punishment, in some manner deserved, or, as St. Paul would have it, that suffering improves character and leads to hope. If hope is the ultimate end, then anything leading to it is meaningful. If I can find a meaning, a reason, then that shelters me and I have much less need to confront and accept reality. The reality that I cannot control the disease activity in my brain, for example, can be obscured if I think that there is meaning and purpose to be found in it.

For some reason the quest for meaning was something I seemed to escape. It never occurred to me to ask why or, more particularly, why me. It happened. It reflected—whatever the etiology of MS turns out to be—a physical event, a malfunctioning of cells. There was no reason why it should not have happened to me. A metaphysical explanation seemed not only irrelevant and unnecessary to me but (assuming I could have come up with a satisfying one) an impediment to full acceptance of present reality. This is what is, it happened to me, and there was not, nor did there need to be, any further meaning. One might ask why I am writing this; is it not a way to give meaning to this experience? Certainly on one level it is, but one of the most important things I have learned is that it is only when one stops trying to find meaning, to assign meaning, that there can be any kind of peace about who and what one is. One of the most difficult aspects of my disease has been the consequences for me of others' need to find meaning in my experience.

I do not believe that there is a moral issue anywhere to be found in the fact that I have multiple sclerosis. Nevertheless, a conflict is created when, overtly or covertly, society in general frames the experience of disease in moral terms. The analogy that comes to mind is the use of the word "atheism"—being defined in terms of that which one believes not to exist. Equally, when disease is framed as a moral issue, it becomes hard to resist.

An incident that illuminated for me many of these values and conflicts—and carried within it these broad themes—occurred at a party, when a friend, in introducing me to a woman, mentioned my MS. As this woman was leaving, she said to me, "You'll be OK; you're a fighter." I was outraged and offended. Beyond the fact that this woman knew nothing about me was the message, given very loudly and clearly, that the outcome of my disease was in my hands; that it was a question ultimately of character; that acceptance is a sign of weakness. The objective reality of the lesions in my brain seemingly have no part to play. She would not have me accept that whether I walk in five years is beyond my control. She would say fight, fight, fight; believe in the illusion that it is within your control and that if you fail, it is because of lack of strength.

I felt very strongly that in her eyes acceptance was equated with weakness, with lack of character. When failure (for I do believe that she would see an inability to walk as a failure) is seen in these terms, as a moral issue, as reflective of a lack of will and character, then denial becomes almost a psychological necessity. For who, after all, wishes to be deemed a moral failure, a loser?

The intensity of my reaction to this woman is, I am sure, explained in part by my experience during the years preceding my diagnosis when, because there was no "good" reason for my recurrent weakness, I was often treated as though I chose to be weak out of some deficiency of character. I know that I overreact in such situations and that, because of my history, I am defensive. Perhaps I hear too loudly the implication that if "it" can be fought, then "it" is in my mind. At moments like that, I see all too clearly that the diagnosis did not resolve the question of legitimacy for me but only changed the terms. I also realize more clearly the continuing importance of resisting others' definition of my experience. The issue of maintaining integrity is not so different even after one has a label.

I do see the achievement of real acceptance as a struggle but that struggle is internal; it does not involve wrestling with immutable facts. There is not an equation between fighting and giving up. Acceptance is more of a process than a goal, and the desired end for me is to reach some equanimity and equilibrium within the context of what cannot be changed and to retain my self throughout that process. Society, in this instance through this woman, tells me to continue to struggle to change the unchangeable. What is important to remember is that I am, whether I like it or not, in the social world and defined by or, perhaps more accurately, set against others' constructs of reality. As with the earlier analogy, there is no word in common usage except "atheist."

What does it mean to be disabled in the face of those assumptions? It was hard enough for me to come to terms with the reality that I have no control over this disease and no knowledge of how, when, or if it will progress. I have learned to live with some ease (with continuing setbacks in that regard) with who I am and the changes imposed by the fact of multiple sclerosis. It seems in some ways that if I were somehow an isolated entity, me and my disease, I could live with more ease. But, of course, that is facile and I am not isolated. I am a part of my society, my experience and my self are affected by it. How does one maintain integrity, a sense of wholeness, in the face of these assumptions, which not only distort one's experience but make acceptance of one's situation very difficult?

The integrity of the person, his or her boundedness, is a Western notion. It might be interesting (although outside my purposes) to consider whether or to what degree the values I have been discussing are a logical outgrowth of this vision of a person as a discrete, self-defined entity. Or whether self as we think of it is a reflection, or a necessary corollary, of these ideas about the nature of reality.

Control over nature, the lack of inherent goodness, autonomy, the centrality of doing, the idea that anything is possible together with the importance of the future—its potential for change—all form a complex within which it would seem that ideally an individual acting autonomously can through the exercise of will and discipline not only control his or her experience but direct it in such a way that the future will inevitably be an improvement. The necessary corollary of all this is that failure is deserved; if these ideas are held to be true and valid notions about the nature of reality, then individual failure (failure to be what one could, should, be?) necessarily reflects defects in character and will.

In my view, the central issue and the continuing task for anyone with a chronic disease is acceptance. It encompasses everything, and its absence—reflected by denial—is also encompassing. The primary cultural values and assumptions taken together (and they are related) all militate against acceptance. If I believe that my MS is a physical event over which I have no control; if I live my life in terms of its given realities and do not rely on hope of change; if I acknowledge that I can do very little about it and more, that who I am is not dependent on what I do; if, finally, I manage to accept that I am not independent— responsible for myself, yes, but clearly unable to live autonomously—then I live at odds with the dominant thrust of my culture.

Self-responsibility, autonomy, material success, and independence are highly valued in American culture. They have been a central part of the American ethos since the country was first settled by Europeans. Reinforced by the Protestant work ethic and Horatio Alger myths, America itself has been symbolic of the notion that with hard work, determination, and a commitment to success, anything is possible for an individual. And, of course, enough people have achieved success in terms commonly recognized as such to keep this dream alive. It is alive for many individuals and also for the country. There is a very strong belief that one can do whatever one wants to do. Many people believe that if you are hungry or poor or unemployed, it is because you simply have not tried hard enough. As a society, we do not want to hear that determination may not be enough; that there are realities that cannot be changed through effort. The poor boy making good through nothing but his own initiative and hard work remains a powerful symbol even in the face of widespread unemployment and hardship. Intuitively, it seems that symbols would lose their power when they overtly conflict with reality, but perhaps they become more powerful than ever.

We, as a society, take great pride in our generosity, our openness. Those who are unable to work, however, are supported at barely subsistence levels. We proclaim the value of work and its rewards, yet there are millions who work full-time and fail to earn enough to raise them out of poverty. Hard work for them does not lead to success. This is an example of an idea that is central to the way in which we perceive ourselves, yet which, in reality, has little to do with the way in which we live, as a nation and as individuals. This kind of conflict has a lot to do with the experience of being chronically ill in this culture. Chronic illness brings one face to face with the conflicts inherent in the underlying structural themes of American culture. One is no longer able to believe in many of the things that are so central to the way in which we perceive ourselves.

Why was the destruction of the Challenger space shuttle such an enormous shock to the American public? We believe that we can do anything, that there are no limits, that strength and will and determination conquer all obstacles. We have an unbridled faith in our ability to do whatever it is we set out to do. The space shuttle disaster is a good example of what we do to avoid seeing limits. We do not want to know that our technological ability is limited; that accidents can and do happen. While with the wisdom of hindsight it seems that this accident might well have been prevented if better judgment had been exercised along the way, the discussion seems to turn on just that point—focusing on individual failures in leadership and judgment. There has been very little acknowledgment that in enterprises of this nature accidents are inevitable.

As a society, we believe that control is possible on both an individual and a social level. Outcomes can be controlled. Results can be determined. Failure is always the result of a lack of will, of determination, ultimately of character. Seen in these terms, failure can bring nothing else than a moral judgment. We, as a group, do not generally acknowledge limits or see any failure as a simple coming up against reality.

The anger of those closest to me when confronted with the fact of my disease is also reflective of this very powerful assumption that control is possible and desirable. I think it is primarily because of the pervasiveness of this belief that, for example, Nick's anger was so extreme. I was sick and there was absolutely nothing he could do about it, yet his instinctive response was to take action, and this response came out of a belief that there is always something that can be done, that action is the appropriate response. To acknowledge lack of control, of the power to change things, is terrifying in its implications. We are not used to doing so. We tend to go to great lengths to avoid it. To do otherwise would involve coming to terms with the ways in which our most cherished beliefs about ourselves and our culture conflict with reality.

The values of control and independence are closely related. If it is important to believe that one is independent and self-sufficient, then one almost has to believe that one can control one's life. Conversely, if control is possible, so is independence. If I am independent and self-sufficient and believe I can control my life, then anything is possible. To admit that there are things that are not possible, things that cannot be changed, would bring the whole edifice tumbling down. I could no longer believe I am in control and would thus be incapable of maintaining the fiction of my independence and self-sufficiency.

I am reminded of an acquaintance with MS who travels all over the world in search of a cure. She spends thousands of dollars on patently sham treatments. She won't see a doctor, however, because "they won't do anything for me, they can't help me" and she cannot acknowledge that an answer is unavailable.

The scene at the airport in Luxor that I described earlier perfectly captures for me the working out of these values. That scene's starkness as a metaphor arises out of contrast—a small group of people actively creating their own world governed by classically American values set down in the midst of a diametrically different culture.

I have been forced to accept that I have no control over—and no knowledge of—the course of this disease; that is a fact and one that I would ignore only at my peril. My psychological and emotional well-being depends on my having come to terms with the fact that I cannot control what happens to me, that no amount (and I don't claim all that much) of strength and determination is going to affect my ability to walk. Those old Americans in Luxor would have me deny that. They would have me believe that I do have control and that the outcome is dependent on my reserves of determination and will and strength.

It is partly because of this belief that, as I have said, in a very hidden, unacknowledged way, illness and disease are seen in moral, not physical, terms. Disease does exist. It cannot be comfortably acknowledged or given a place within this broad cultural framework. It must be seen as somehow anomalous. The answer is to see disease and disability as a moral outcome and as a punishment even while we profess to view it scientifically. This makes it possible, if what is seen as a desired outcome is not achieved, to believe that it results from lack of will, lack of determination.

While acceptance carries with it the implication of weakness in this culture, denial connotes strength, a fighting against, a refusal to give in. Therein lies a conflict. The primary task—and the most difficult—facing anyone with a chronic disease is acceptance. It encompasses everything else. But, as I have tried to show, the most basic and deeply held values and assumptions of this culture militate against acceptance. If I accept the full implications of the realities imposed by the fact of my multiple sclerosis, I am living in conflict with those values. If I accept what I think I must accept, I am judged and found wanting by society. I come up squarely against the most important cultural myths and assumptions. My disease reflects the imperfection of my nature; it indicates a lack of control where we need and would like to believe that we have control; it forces me to believe that tomorrow will not necessarily be better; it is something I can "do" nothing about; and it calls into question my autonomy and independence.

The assumptions that seemed to me to be paramount and controlling in the books about MS—the emphasis on physical factors and responses, the reliance on hope, the seemingly essential optimism—are not only explicable but inevitable once one considers the cultural frame. I think it becomes clear that as acceptance is an encompassing umbrella for what is necessary to adjust to chronic disease, so denial encompasses the range of responses that would be, broadly speaking, culturally acceptable. It is those responses, consequently, that are emphasized in most books about MS. For example, the emphasis on physical factors in most of what I read seems clearly to be both a result of and a response to the cultural values I have identified. If one believes that only physical adjustment is necessary, then one is both reflecting the imperatives of this culture and denying their deeper implications.

I feel as though I am continually faced by the judgment that my disability is a moral outcome, not an objective reality. If I were to deny the implications of my disease, were to struggle and fight against the reality of my disability, were to rely on hope as a response and a way out, I would be more in tune with my culture and would be viewed in a more favorable light by most people.

This, then, is the cultural framework—very broadly and superficially drawn—within which the experience of chronic illness fits or does not fit. The primary themes—self-determination, individualism, materialism—do structure experience. It is important to realize that even as individuals hold other values to be paramount or feel themselves to be outside or beyond the reach of the world shaped by these values, they are still subject to and influenced by that framework—as the nature and shape of a counterculture is bound to be dominated, if not determined, by the nature of the culture to which it is a reaction.

I think that all of these factors and the reasons for them explain, at least in part, my sense of comfort and ease in the Middle East. This is a very superficial reading of another culture, but I think it was, in essence, the sense one has in Egypt that what has happened has happened, what will happen will happen, that was so congruent with my understanding and acceptance of what has happened to me and made being there so very easy and comfortable for me. Here almost everything conflicts to a greater or lesser degree with my intuitive understanding of what I need to do and be to live with this disease.

Acceptance and living without hope, as I envision it, do not mean living in despair. Rather, it means looking at one's life and the range of possible outcomes with clear eyes. When I look at myself and my life without illusion, without false hope of change, then and only then can I live fully and positively. I think there is great freedom and a rare kind of peace to be found in acceptance that, for me at any rate, is essential.

I realize, on reading this, that I have conveyed the impression that life, for me, is a constant battle. That is certainly not the case. There are many days and many ways in which the fact of my MS is not relevant to my daily life. But there is also a very real and omnipresent way in which I feel that the society I live in would like to ignore the realities of my life and, barring that, would have me ignore them so that I am not an affront to other people's sensibilities and more, do not cause them to question the basic underpinnings of their vision of the nature of reality. I can accept the disease or I can accept the dominant values of this society; I doubt it is possible to do both.

American culture is not going to change significantly—at least in my lifetime—and I will continue to be a part of American society. It was crucial for me to try to understand the cultural framework within which I live in order to comprehend why people act the way they do. The more I understand the elements that structure my experience, the easier it is to come to terms with it. Understanding is essential to acceptance.

# Uncertainty and Process

Before I could look at my experience within that cultural framework, it very slowly became clear to me that there were two essential facets of the experience of chronic illness that had to be fully explored. In that exploration, the sense of forward progress and of momentum ceases. These issues require both time out, as it were, and a realization that they will continue to be issues and will, in the end, fail to be resolved.

The first issue is absolutely central and affects my responses to and thinking about all the others. It is difficult to formulate; nevertheless, I will try because I begin to think that it is crucial to the entire process of acceptance and adjustment. Moreover, I think that on the level of daily life it is enormously important. It was a long time before I was fully aware of this issue and I am still not sure what to call it—a sense of generalized vulnerability perhaps, an unsureness or uncertainty.

One reason why it took so long to become aware of this was because the diagnosis was such a powerful event for me. It had, in retrospect, wiped out the doubt and uncertainty I had had during those fourteen years before I knew I had MS. My perceptions had been affirmed and my uncertainty erased by a fact. I perceived the diagnosis, that moment of clarity, as not only reaching back to transform the past but as carrying me through the future. It gave me, and my experience, a solid underpinning and affirmation. It took time before I let go of that solid fact enough to see that there was a completely new kind of uncertainty that was affecting me.

This new uncertainty arises from the site of this disease. I stumble, limp, drop things, but there is nothing wrong with my arms or legs as such. The disease process and the resulting damage is in my brain. This fact raises questions for me that, while imperative, are also unanswerable (at least at present). What is my self? What are its boundaries and where is it to be found? What is it that makes me who I am and what of that is essential? Will I know if I cease to be who I am? It seems unlikely because I would no longer be there to know it. How does my self know itself?

All of this posits and assumes a dichotomy between my body and my mind (or, is it more properly, self?)—a separation. The two are not the same. I do not feel that my body is congruent with my self. And beyond that, while on one level I seem to be saying that self and brain do have some congruence, on another level, that is also unclear. Certainly, in some ways I feel my self to be at stake vis-à-vis my body. In others, I equally clearly do not.

This distinction troubles me because of its inherent (or are they?) metaphysical implications to which I do not subscribe. But certainly on an operational level, I do see my body as something apart from and indeed, at times, as alien to me. I see my self as having an independent existence. But I do see my self and my brain as being inextricably entwined.

This is all very problematic and culture-bound. But I am a product of my culture and this is my bias. It is intriguing to speculate about (and of course, impossible to know) exactly how one might feel if one did not have this dualistic view. If I felt no distinction, no separation, between body and self, would I feel more or less threatened by bodily malfunctions? Remembering how I felt on those days when, because of ACTH, I failed to recognize myself, I think if I had really felt that my body was me, I might have felt the loss of self. But this is idle speculation; I at least cannot enter fully into the imagination of a wholly other. I can only realize the ways in which my imaginative vision may be colored and distorted; the distortion can never be entirely removed.

I mentioned earlier the awe I felt looking at the CT scan showing the lesions in my brain. My damaged brain observing the damage in my brain. How can I trust that observation?

Should I? What of my thoughts about the world, about the nature of reality, my perceptions and judgments of people and events—are they to be trusted? I wonder, writing this, whether there is coherence and sense to be found here.

An uncertainty at the very center of me. Where are "the neural foundations of the self" to be found?[1] Will I develop a lesion that will irrevocably change the essence of my self? An unscientific notion, perhaps, but still a thought that in the stillness of the night recurs. And even more sobering, if that were to happen, would I know or would I continue to trust the integrity of my self?

These questions pose an existential quandary that is very real for me. If my leg and my arm were in fact damaged, these thoughts would not arise, my self would not be at stake. (If I were an athlete, of course, it might well be.) It is precisely the fact that my self does seem in some measure to be at issue that, I think, both complicates enormously the process of thinking clearly about some issues—for example, the whole question of strength and weakness—and makes them even more important. Seeing the culture clearly and my experience set against that backdrop has some illuminating power in this context.

Of a slightly different order but clearly linked to this uncertainty is a physical wariness that is new to me. I often hesitate now to do things that I used to think little of, and yet I always wonder whether I overreact. I feel more vulnerable in a physical way but it is not primarily a physical issue. I find that I second-guess myself ever more frequently and on all levels. I spoke of some of this earlier. My wariness is clearly related to the unknown course of the disease. With time, I find it seems even more important that I achieve some clarity about the consequences of this uncertainty. The world of relationships and of motivation is murky enough and complex enough. I do not want the fact of this disease and its effect on me to add yet another layer of undifferentiated confusion. It seems crucial that I at least be aware of how my self and my behavior are affected by

1. Oliver Sacks, *The Man Who Mistook His Wife for a Hat* (New York: Summit Books, 1985), p. xiv.

this sense of vulnerability and uncertainty. I am who I am but is my perception of that always trustworthy? Are my actions or responses always reasonable or, indeed, appropriate?

The effects of stress contribute to this generalized uncertainty. I mentioned that I am apt to become confused in extreme heat; I may not act or respond rationally, and during that time of confusion I may not know that I am confused. (I have learned that much; have I missed something else? Am I confused without knowing I am confused?) A damaged central nervous system, I am told, does not handle stress as well as it might; it overloads faster, it does not process stress efficiently or correctly. I know from experience that in situations of extreme stress (and not so extreme—what is extreme for me now is not what used to be) I do not function very well.

While I have learned quite a bit about what causes stress and how much is too much, my knowledge remains inexact and entirely too variable for any comfort or certainty. There are days when I can do almost anything; there are also days when, for no discernible reason, I am absolutely and suddenly exhausted. And it is, of course, this real and physical uncertainty that contributes to the greater uncertainty. The result is an inchoate but very definite and pervasive sense of uncertainty and vulnerability. There are, as always, different levels at which this uncertainty operates. At its most basic, for example, I always wonder, if I drive to a place two hours away, whether I will be able to get back. More generally, how trustworthy are my perceptions of and reactions to people and events? This should not be overstated; nevertheless, it is very real and does, I know, affect my approach and response to all of life.

Because this heightened sense of vulnerability does affect me in this fashion, when I am thinking about an issue such as dependency I tend to wonder whether I am too sensitive to it or see it as larger than it is. What is important is that all of my experience and my perception of the conflicts raised by the fact of having MS is filtered through or informed by that sense of uncertainty. It is necessary to recognize this, although by its very nature and diffuseness, I am never quite sure of the degree to which or in quite what fashion this uncertainty operates. It is also clear that perhaps because of the nature of uncertainty, many of these thoughts have no clear ending point. The fact that there may be no intellectually satisfying resolution does not in itself make the process unnecessary or unfruitful. These quandaries, notwithstanding their essential elusiveness, have been and remain a central part of this entire experience for me.

Thinking about my life seen through this filter, I have wondered how it would have been different had I not known that I have MS. I have spoken of the uncertainty I felt before I knew I had multiple sclerosis—uncertainty both before and after the diagnosis. The old uncertainty arose from lack of knowledge. The new comes precisely from that knowledge I so ardently desired. There is irony there. I would always choose to have that knowledge, however. Without it, I would have had to continue to wrestle with a phantom. My close relationships would have continued to be flawed by that lack of trust I spoke of. And I wonder whether, with time, I might have become quite thoroughly depressed and neurotic and lost the ability to continue to insist on the essential rightness of my own perceptions.

As being in the Middle East illuminated for me the broad impact of culture on my experience, so did thinking about what happened to me the day I received my diagnosis prove illuminating vis-à-vis personal reality. It provided a glimpse of both the social reality of disease and the social construction of that reality. How did that knowledge, the reception of a diagnosis, change my life? Objectively, nothing changed; subjectively, everything changed. I did not change on the day I received the diagnosis. The social consequences for me were altered, which in turn altered the subjective quality of my experience. I entered a new social world, the world of disease. I think I saw that world more clearly and certainly faster because of all those years of not knowing and living with the consequences of that. But it was also because I did so clearly see the diagnosis as a central event, one that would provide resolution, that I more quickly saw its limitations. It eventually became clear to me that structurally some of the elements of my experience, before and after the diagnosis, were very similar. The reasons for and the nature of my uncertainty, for example, were very different; yet the uncertainty continues. And, as before, so after, I could only try to live my own life. The phantom was revealed as a very concrete reality. Now I wrestle with fact and with the social world and its construction of disease.

What is interesting to me in retrospect is exactly how dramatically my experience was altered by receiving a diagnosis, a label. I was radically transformed that day; it was not only that others' perceptions changed, my own perspective on my experience changed. And certainly others' perception of me did change. Behavior that was illegitimate when I was "well" was suddenly legitimate when I was "sick." There was power in that social reality—mediated and experienced through the culture and cultural values—to form and shape my individual experience. My history was in a sense altered, it retrospectively changed. But what really happened? Nothing happened. I was given (as were others) a label and a new filter through which to view my experience. Over the years I had been sick without being so labeled; my ability to function had been impaired without an accepted and legitimizing reason. Now, suddenly, there was a label, attached retroactively, which seemed retrospectively to alter relationships and history.

It seems useful to look at the conflicts I experience and attempt to resolve through that filter—the overlay, as it were, which so definitively changed everything. Nothing changed that day and everything changed. I was vindicated and affirmed. From being in an anomalous situation, suddenly I was categorized. It was not the knowledge in and of itself; the knowledge that there was a discrete reason for all that happened to me was comforting but it did not change my physical reality. My understanding, and that of others, of my condition changed. A diagnosis, a reason, altered perceptions and judgments; it irrevocably changed the environment within which I live. Of course, the physical consequences of the disease were much easier to bear in the framework of that knowledge. Before the diagnosis, I was always being told that any symptoms I experienced were a result of my own behavior or of neurosis; and an inevitable part of that was that if I was sick, it was my own fault. That was hard to bear and ultimately, hard to resist. Those fourteen years between what my neurologist now thinks was the onset of my MS and its diagnosis were a long time.

Receiving a diagnosis was, as I said, an act of affirmation. My perceptions and intuitions about what had happened to me had been, in fact, correct. More essentially, the prism changed. And that process, an abrupt change of lenses as it were, allowed a glimpse of the social construction of disease. From that day forward, my experience, which in some ways remained the same, was structured by a quite different set of cultural expectations and norms, and thus its quality as well as its shape was altered. But the clarity I expected to continue was in many ways an illusion.

The second essential facet of the experience of chronic illness became clear to me exactly as I began to recognize the illusive nature of that clarity. Clarity fades in and out precisely because of the nature of acceptance. Acceptance is commonly seen as an event and I, at first, perceived the achieving of acceptance as a track on which *A* led inevitably to *Z*. Indeed, in the first few years after my diagnosis, there was a clear and fairly speedy progression from the shock I spoke of to an acceptance of the fact of the disease. But that rock-bottom acceptance is really only a prologue to living that acceptance. What I see as the crucial point about acceptance, and the most misunderstood, becomes the salient reality—that acceptance is a process and, in no sense, an event. What acceptance means in daily life is a constantly changing, evolving, and sometimes messy reality. The sense of progress ceases and one is left with the true nature of acceptance as I see it; its essence is process. There is no end, no point at which one can say, "Aha! I have accepted. On to the next task." What is involved in living acceptance is processual[2] and, indeed, repetitive. Continuing and maintaining acceptance requires an ongoing series of changes, refinements, even realizations. The remainder of this story is very reflective of my understanding that acceptance is a process. The experience and thus the telling of it is to a degree repetitive, even circular; it is much slower-paced, as was the living.

2. Processual is not to be found in a dictionary; nonetheless, it seems the best word to describe what I wish to describe.

The uncertainty I speak of here is a good example of this. One can and does accept that one lives and will live in great and continuing uncertainty. The basic fact of the uncertainty is sooner or later accepted. The playing out of uncertainty, its realization and meaning in daily life, is continuous. I continue to become aware of the implications of that uncertainty for me, its impact on relationships, and on large and small decisions. The consequences of that uncertainty continue to unfold.

With the passage of time it becomes ever more clear to me that acceptance is not discrete and certainly neither a state nor a static condition. It is a task but not one that can be completed and marked as achieved. I stress this because I find people generally and, it sometimes seems to me, almost obstinately, misunderstand acceptance.

The common understanding of acceptance, perhaps arising out of a simplistic reading of Elisabeth Kubler-Ross's work on stages, is seriously flawed. Acceptance is commonly seen as the final event in a series of stages. Whether or not Kubler-Ross intended that is open to question, but the result is that acceptance is generally seen as a discrete event, an achievable task. This is quite wrong. One might perhaps more usefully perceive acceptance as that which makes the working out of acceptance, its living, possible. Words fail me here. Acceptance that one has a chronic disease is, indeed, essential but what that really means is a continuing realization and acknowledgment of its consequences.

I accept that I have MS; what having MS means for me on a daily basis, however, is a continually changing reality. In my closest relationships, for example, the fact that I have a chronic disease continues to have new effects and consequences. Without the bottom-line acceptance, I couldn't begin to accept—primarily because I would not see—the myriad ways in which my disease affects these relationships.

There is another aspect of acceptance that I think is open to great misunderstanding. Acceptance does not preclude moments of despair or moments of feeling totally at sea or of wanting to hide, nor does acceptance preclude anger. Such moments do not call acceptance into question. I think there is a prevailing notion that acceptance does away with conflict and anger.

My growing understanding that living with MS, or any chronic disease in this society, inevitably places one in a position of continuing conflict is an example of this. I do not feel that acceptance necessarily or even usually obviates those conflicts but rather that part of what acceptance involves is an acknowledgment of those conflicts and of the reality that they will continue, albeit realized and experienced in ever-changing ways. Understanding the roots of those conflicts is essential to acceptance but acceptance neither negates the conflicts nor robs them of their importance.

On a more personal level, acceptance does not mean that there will not be problems or that there will not be anger (on my part or the part of a lover or spouse); acceptance is rather what provides the possibility of integrating the fact of the disease into a life. Both the reality and the circumstances of my life continue to change, and that continuing reality requires continuing clarity as one recognizes and confronts the new effects and consequences of MS.

It has become increasingly clear to me that there is a very widespread reluctance to acknowledge even the possibility of negative feelings in a relationship in which one partner has a chronic disease. There seems to be a notion floating around that acknowledging anger or acknowledging that both partners will occasionally feel anger or resentment calls the entire relationship into question; that "true" acceptance would preclude any negative feelings. This is naïve in the extreme. It is crucial to recognize that in a relationship where one person is continually physically needy there are almost bound to be times when both resent this, regardless of the underlying strength and soundness of the relationship.

In fact, I think the stronger and sounder the relationship, the more apt each person is to express negative feelings. It is only in a relationship based on complete honesty and acceptance that one can easily and openly express anger. Openly acknowledging and expressing these feelings is essential. We are none of us saints. Acceptance, on my part and on the part of my spouse or lover, is exactly what allows the expression of anger. Anger is not a bad thing. It is often the way we express feelings such as resentment or frustration. I tend to think it is more efficient of time and energy to identify what causes the anger before it reaches the anger stage; nevertheless, in practice, I think we often find ourselves angry and only then identify the reason.

Beyond that, it is crucial to understand that acceptance of the disease does not, will not, and I don't think in the end necessarily should preclude anger at some of its consequences. The consequences continue to unfold. They are not immediately apparent. I am reminded of a moment that I hold in my mind as illustrative of this dynamic, a first canoe ride with a friend. We were paddling along and a moment came when I realized I could no longer hold that paddle with my left arm, much less continue to paddle. I knew that I had to tell him that he would have to paddle on that side. Of course, given the nature of canoes, he would have soon realized this in any event. Telling him was exceedingly difficult for me; I felt anger, dismay, and resentment at the physical reality that I could no longer continue to paddle, at the fact that I had to deal with the situation at all, at the fact that obviously I would not be an ideal person with whom to undertake a long canoe trip. All kinds of thoughts and emotions flashed through my mind at that moment before I forced myself to speak to him. The conflicts I felt were present despite the fact that I felt completely accepted and that my weakness is clearly not an issue in this relationship. Of course, I did tell him, and he, having no idea of what I had been thinking, said sure, and we sailed on. The moment and the difficulty were all mine. I think my anger and dismay in that situation arose precisely out of my acceptance. Had I not accepted the fact of the disease, I would not have seen that moment as yet another unfolding of the meaning of acceptance. It was the acceptance that forced me to acknowledge that particular consequence and my anger (dismay) arose out of the knowledge that here was yet another circumstance that required adjustment—a perfect example of acceptance as process.

The dictionary meanings of "acceptance" include "accommodation or reconciliation of oneself to something" and "endurance." Both accommodation and endurance carry implications of process. I certainly get tired of this process, and part of my frustration in that moment arose precisely out of my continuing realization that the consequences and the unfolding of my acceptance were a never-to-be-ended process. I had never thought about canoes. I would have liked very much to be able to paddle for hours with ease and no thought. I think that a failure to accept that frustration as a natural response or a requirement to pretend that such moments do not sometimes give rise to anger and frustration is very self-defeating. This notion that acceptance precludes conflict or anger is clearly related to the emphasis on hope and optimism I spoke of earlier. I think there is a belief that both acceptance and hope should make the existence (not to mention the expression) of negative feelings impossible. This, of course, leads right back into denial and I do believe there is a large element of denial operating in common understandings of acceptance. It is important to recognize that experiencing anger and frustration is a way in which we do live acceptance; it is, perhaps, even essential.

My moment in the canoe is an example also of the repetitive and often circular process that acceptance both is and requires. Acceptance does not do away with the need to become aware of a new consequence of disease in a relationship, for example, and to come to terms with it and integrate it into the relationship. Of course, my canoe ride is a very concrete and limited example of something that is usually much more important, diffuse, and difficult. It is in such new situations that we recapitulate, consolidate, and live true acceptance. I knew at that moment that what was going through my mind was not new. It was in many ways a repetition of similar situations in the past. Each new unfolding is quicker because it holds within it past experience; nevertheless, it is unique.

The issue of uncertainty and the notion of acceptance as process are clearly related. More important, they are very similar kinds of issues, both in their centrality and in their open-endedness. Becoming aware of some of the implications of uncertainty and acceptance was necessary to begin to understand some of the more concrete consequences of chronic illness.

Just as my understanding of the social and cultural conflicts that chronic illness gives rise to did not obviate those conflicts, so understanding does not do away with conflict in daily life or in a relationship. Understanding is essential to acceptance but there is no closure. Acceptance of and adjustment to a life lived in the frame of chronic disease will never be completed. Forward momentum may cease; widening and deepening (or is it consolidation) never ends.

# Chronically Ill in America

*Illness is the night-side of life,*
*a more onerous citizenship.*
SUSAN SONTAG

The clarity provided by the diagnosis does, of course, remain and its power to affirm me as an individual was real. But as I gained some understanding of the ways in which the chronically ill are affected by American values, I began to see more clearly the limits of that clarity and that event that had so much power for me. The values that underlie American culture are a central part of the framework within which I live and within which disease and disability must fit, however awkwardly. The social and cultural conflicts I described earlier are, in a sense, general. The more specific individual conflicts are framed by those values; one cannot live a life shaped by disease without becoming aware that its reality is in conflict with the general thrust of this culture.

My experience has been and continues to be shaped and colored by living within this world view. Certainly, as I said, it is not an omnipresent battle, but it does underlie my experience. Seeing that larger context eased the process of coming to terms with what MS meant to me. Knowledge is not explanation but it is necessary. I do in the end remain who I am beyond anyone's definition, but it is easy to forget that. Understanding the cultural dynamics eases the process.

Once I had some awareness of this cultural framework and its impact on the diseased and disabled, the controversy about language began to make some intuitive sense to me as reflecting the impact of the primary values of this culture on the disabled.

I began to understand some of what lies behind this often heated debate about language. Clearly there is a level at which it is irrelevant. So I am now a cripple or disabled or handicapped. All of those words are labels and not very useful ones. They convey little information beyond stereotypical images. I still find it difficult to think the choice of words matters very much, but I do begin to understand what lies behind the debate.

The words in and of themselves are very interesting, as is the continuing controversy over their use. There is some information about the social reality of disease to be found in these words. One source says, "Being handicapped is a social term with negative connotations which foster images of helplessness."[1] The preferred term is "disabled." I went to the dictionary and discovered that "disabled" means "incapacitated by illness" and a disability is an "inability to pursue an occupation because of physical or mental impairment." A "cripple" is a "lame or partly disabled person" and, secondarily, "something flawed or imperfect." A "handicap" is "a disadvantage that makes achievement unusually difficult."

Given these definitions, I prefer "handicapped" or even "crippled." Either word is both more accurate and more pointed. "Disabled" or "disability" has more of a legal connotation. But all of the fuss over nomenclature is another example of the social/cultural attitudes which impede adjustment to a disease such as MS. I am handicapped. I am not exactly like a healthy person. Just as in a horse race, I am carrying more weight (in a manner of speaking) and, therefore, I use more energy to go the same distance. That is a reality. If one is less able to manage, why the imperative to deny it with euphemistic and ever vaguer expressions? "Images of helplessness"—why? And beyond that, why, if one does need help, is that need viewed so negatively?

But, of course, I find that this line of thought does inevitably circle round; I see it in myself. No, I am not the same as everyone else and I often wish there was some acknowledgment of that fact. On a bad day, it would be nice if someone noticed how

1. Judith McLaughlin, "Multiplying the Health Potential of the Person with Multiple Sclerosis," *Health Values* 10, no. 4 (July/August 1986): 17.

very hard it can be for me just to be at work. On the other hand, I do want to be seen as acceptable, as whole, and not as "other than." Even when I objectively need help, I resist asking for it.

I think the dislike of the word "handicapped" is indicative of this conflict—a desire to be treated at one and the same time as both different and as the same. The preferred (if unlikely) outcome, of course, is for the other to make it possible for that to happen. In many ways it is I, the culture working through and reflected in me, who negatively loads the words and creates the conflicts. The culture is not only an external operating force. If I were an alien, would I feel these conflicts at all? Perhaps, but not perhaps in the same way.

The Special Olympics is a good example of this—different and yet the same. The event expresses competition, the need to excel and win, to demonstrate endurance—a desire to show that the disabled are driven by, the same forces and values as everyone else. It demonstrates the values of the culture writ plain, albeit in a very protected environment. It might also be said that institutions such as the Special Olympics provide an opportunity for participants to live up to their potential, unhindered by external, artificial constraints. However, it remains an example of an attempt to ignore the fact that the handicapped are different.

I think the issue of the handicapped's access to public facilities comes in here, too. While I have become very sensitive to that issue and know that I may be in a wheelchair one day, I have real difficulty in accepting the notion that society should bear the enormous cost involved in making all facilities accessible to the handicapped. As I see it, however, all of this—language, institutions such as the Special Olympics, the access question—represents a blurring and a reflection of the desire on the part of both society and the handicapped individual to create a situation in which people are the same, or to pretend that they are. It is also a way to both deny and, on one level, deal with some of the conflicts raised.

We do not, in this culture, deal easily or well with the weak and dependent. We are not straightforward; we view these conditions through the mist of our values. We see them not as purely physical and objective conditions but as reflecting, in part, a moral issue. Weakness *is* a metaphor for failure; we *do* see weakness in terms of failure. Metaphor both creates and reflects social reality; it organizes experience. But we are not honest about this response. To mask this, language must be misused, boundaries blurred. We do the same thing with death.

Of course, beyond the culture and beyond words, I am who I am and in some essential way remain beyond the reach of the judgments of others. There always remains a sense in which those judgments are not relevant to me. But those judgments, equally, are what I am talking about. It is because I feel that physical weakness is often seen as moral weakness that it becomes difficult to accept. Rarely is there a sense that weakness is a legitimate response and thus, for the individual, giving in, even accepting, becomes an internal question of some magnitude. Why else do I insist on my essential OK-ness and accept in some way as my own other people's definition of that? Why else do children compete in the Special Olympics if not to prove that they, too, hold as central, and are driven by the same values as the rest of the populace? This is an intensely competitive, success-oriented, and materialistic society. But those values are not my values and those judgments cease to be of consequence at some level. Life at its most basic, at its center, is untouched. Nonetheless, I do live with and within the prevalent value system of this culture. I have found through my experience with MS that I cannot remain aloof from or untouched by the consequences of this value structure for those who through disease or disability are placed at odds with the general thrust of this culture.

Beyond generalities, what of daily life? The issues and conflicts that more directly shape and impinge on my day-to-day life arise in large measure out of these values and can clearly be traced to them. These more daily conflicts and issues are, in some ways, subsidiary to the larger conflicts I identified and are certainly less abstract. With time I realized that most of what is most problematic for me is subsumed by the issue of dependence and the strength/weakness dilemma. These conflicts became clearer and to a degree more manageable when I saw them as resulting from the cultural system as a whole; I could then place them in a larger framework and begin to understand them.

Again, to the degree that this process of acceptance and adjustment appears repetitive and circular, it is because it both was and is. The initial shock and adjustments to the fact that I had a chronic disease were, I think, necessarily very personal. Even the impact on my relationships and the adjustments required by that impact were initially intensely personal. It was not until I had reached a new level of equilibrium and moved out into the world, so to speak, that I became aware of how significantly my diagnosis had altered the social terrain for me. Far from resolving everything, the terms of the struggle to maintain integrity had merely shifted—from the personal to the social and cultural.

Once that became clear to me, it was also apparent that there was far more to acceptance than I had thought. As I began to understand the broader implications of being sick in this culture and began to see that more was required than acceptance and adjustment on a personal level, I had to go back. Before I could really come to terms with the issue of dependence, for example, I had to look at it and at myself in the context of those cultural values I talked about. My own adjustment had to incorporate that new understanding. It was not just a personal issue. And so, in a sense, I had to recapitulate those initial adjustments to incorporate those social and cultural aspects.

I have tried to outline some of what underlies and shapes the individual conflicts that seem so crucially important if one is truly to come to terms with and adjust to the full implications of being chronically ill in this culture. These conflicts are complicated by the cultural milieu in which I live; they are further complicated by the sense of uncertainty and vulnerability I tried to elucidate; and, of course, by the particular circumstances of my life, or of anyone's. An issue such as dependence involves all of these factors. Clearly, my own uncertain understanding of dependence or any other conflict is based on my own experience. And, a neurological disorder necessarily invokes fundamental questions of self.

It is, of course, my own experience that has led me to raise these questions. Equally, it is only that experience that I can speak of or from. On the other hand, I wonder if the conclusions I have drawn are generalizable. It is perhaps the structure of my life that has highlighted these issues for me; if my life were different, perhaps their clarity would be obscured. But I do wonder whether my thinking about the experience of chronic illness is so shaped by the particular circumstances of my life as to be idiosyncratic.

I think it is possible that living through those years when I did not know what was wrong with me and, over time, becoming aware of the ways in which that experience affected my relationships enabled me to see more clearly, after the diagnosis, some of the impact of MS on relationships. Because of the experience with not knowing, the effects of knowing were highlighted. My awareness of the impact of the disease on my sense of self-worth, for example, and the implications of the social construction of disease were all perhaps clearer because of those years. I had had time to get used to the need to maintain personal integrity in the face of disbelief and disapprobation, so being faced with the social position that seems to go along with disease and disability in this culture was not so very different. And in many ways, of course, it was much clearer than what had happened to me over all those years.

As I have mentioned, my ex-husband and I are very close. In the years since my diagnosis, he has stood by me in every conceivable way, offering help and support and a kind of love that is very rare. During those years, I had another relationship that was central to me in a different kind of way. Although constrained by circumstances, it was strong, enduring, and sustaining. I am very well loved. Yet neither of those two relationships, for all their importance to me, was complete or very ordinary— in the sense of sharing life in all its dailiness. I spent much time alone during those years and that solitude was important; it forced me to come to terms with my fears and to see my dependence, real and potential, starkly and in relief against those relationships. I think that my solitude, together with those two relationships, so central and yet each incomplete, gave me a clarity that otherwise might have taken me longer to achieve. The dynamics were clear.

I think there is a sense in which I became more quickly aware of some of the implications of chronic disease for relationships because of these circumstances than if I had been in a more conventional marriage or relationship. These two relationships were voluntary, as it were; I have always been aware that being with me even at my neediest has been a choice rather than a requirement following on a commitment made in ignorance. I am always very aware, for example, that what is given is a gift; there is no framework of custom or duty which mandates the help that is offered. My sometime discomfort at receiving (or is it needing?) help is also highlighted by these circumstances.

If I were, it sometimes seems, in a marriage bound and informed by a stated commitment, I would more likely expect a certain level of support and help and might not see the dynamics involved so clearly. I think perhaps the inevitable resentment and anger might be more hidden and my awareness of exactly what is being given and asked for might be diminished. It is also possible that, within a marriage, my husband would feel so trapped and obligated that he would be unable to see how much of what he gave was, in fact, a gift.

Those who are closest to me have also had to come to terms with and accept the possibility of my dependence. It was a long time before I saw this from their point of view—my level of self-absorption was fairly high. Suddenly, they were faced with the real possibility of a future never before conceived. And just as I did, those who love me best have to come to terms with that.

Fear, my own and another's, is another part of this complex that I think I have seen more clearly in these circumstances. Just as the fact of a marriage might obscure the reality of what is given and what is asked for, so I think it might make it harder to acknowledge the fear that is an inevitable part of a disease such as MS. I have found it very easy in these two relationships to be open about my fears. That may well be a reflection of the nature of those men or those relationships but I intuitively feel that the presence of a legal tie might inhibit the expression, on both sides, of fear of what might happen and that the resulting denial would have devastating consequences.

Nick and I are divorced, and we have not discussed in depth all the implications of my potentially increasing dependence. I know that if I am in need, he will help me if he is able. The importance of that knowledge is enormous. And over the years he has lived with my weakness. Perhaps the very absence of a legal tie robs the question of much of its potency. What he offers, and it is ongoing and significant, is clearly a gift, freely given.

The other man I love and I have discussed my potential dependence. What would happen if we were together and I became very ill? This is a hypothetical question and perhaps because of that discussed more freely. I have been moved by his honesty in talking about the whole complex range of feelings and responses that are inevitable over time in a relationship in which one person is physically dependent—the guilt, anger, resentment.

None of what I have said is meant to suggest that I think a marriage relationship cannot absorb and even be strengthened by the presence of chronic illness. But I do think that had I, at least, been married at the time of my diagnosis, it would have taken much longer to achieve clarity about exactly what is at issue. Looking back, I feel very lucky that I had these two extraordinary relationships through which I could see so clearly the impact of my MS. What has been given to me is a gift and in the freedom of those gifts, both the giving and the receiving, there was great clarity.

I feel very strongly, and perhaps wrongly, that with the level of honesty and trust I have known in these two relationships, almost anything is survivable. And that the worst that might happen could be lived with and lived with well if there is that honesty and trust and an openness about what is happening to each other. Dependence puts enormous strain on a relationship and it is complicated both by our own experience of it and by its social construction. We do see it through the filter of those cultural values. But I think it is possible to separate the various structural elements. I can, with some effort, see the distinction between the reality of my dependence in a particular relationship and the ways in which I, and others, tend to overload that reality with common understandings and reactions to dependence. That is essential.

On a personal level, it seems clear that the best one can do is to accept that in a relationship framed by chronic disease there

will be fear, guilt, anger, resentment—on both sides—to be
aware of that possibility, even that certainty, and to openly acknowledge those feelings when they exist. I can think of nothing
worse than sensing the presence of anger and resentment and
not being able to bring those feelings into the open.

For all my talk of acceptance, physical dependence remains
my worst fear, partly because of these inevitable feelings. Despite my understanding, I continue to muddle relationships because of that fear. An example of that is my need for certainty in
my emotional life. I know its roots and I know, too, that there is
no certainty in life. Nevertheless, it gets in my way. All I can do
is hold the awareness of that need in my consciousness and try
not to let it muddle my relationships. A commitment to absolute
honesty, again on both sides, seems essential to me. It is the only
response to a situation that will not go away. During those
years, it was those two so different relationships, set against my
solitude, which helped me to see more clearly than I might otherwise have done some of the consequences of my MS.

The image of the rock that I referred to earlier persists in my
mind. The fact of my MS and, more important, the possibilities
inherent in it is a rock thrown into the pool of all my relationships. There are two outcomes, only one to be desired. The first
is when the stream feeding the pool re-forms around the rock
and new currents and eddies are created so that the rock becomes integrated, a new part of the pool. The other is when the
rock, perhaps too large for that pool, becomes an obstruction—
twigs and leaves are caught up against it and the water begins
to back up. The rock then becomes the dominant element in the
pool and the pool, unable to absorb it and integrate it into its
life, begins to die. Whatever the outcome, that rock is there.

It is out of my own experience that what I have of awareness
and clarity has arisen. Seeing my own culture as an outsider—
in relief—showed me its broad outlines, its structural elements.
The simple, objective, and in itself meaningless act of receiving a diagnosis, illuminated the power that basic assumptions
about reality and common understandings of disease and disability (my own as well as others') have to redefine and alter experience. It is in the daily low-level assumptions that so strongly

color our lives and which flow out of the broader values I talked about earlier that the conflicts I find so central to my life arise.

Once diagnosed, I was suddenly subject to and the object of common knowledge and understandings of disease, common expectations of role behavior, labeling, and the transforming, legitimating, and limiting power of a label. All these factors combined to change my personal reality. Generally speaking, it seems that people do not differentiate between disease and illness or, more particularly, between chronic disease and illness; all ailments are viewed as though they are illnesses. Illness tends to be seen as a discrete episode with a beginning and an end. One recovers or one dies. MS, or chronic disease of any kind, confounds these expectations. I have a disease, I am "disabled" in some ways, and yet I am generally "well." And even on my worst days, I am not "ill" in any conventional sense.

Labeling does occur and it has both positive and negative consequences. Once one is labeled, there is a set of behavior which is explicable and a defined expectation level. I have MS and people, knowing that, accept as natural or inevitable certain consequences. There is a level of explanation that already exists. On the other hand, because of these common understandings of disease, there are many who insist on treating me as sick and who try to force me to conform to their understanding of that role. There are also those who, because I do not fit their understanding of what being sick means, refuse to acknowledge that I may be limited in any way.

When I was first diagnosed I had great difficulty with all of this. I often felt—regardless of which side of this equation someone was on—that *I* was forgotten. It seemed to me then that people looked at me and saw MS and, depending upon their understanding of MS and what it meant, reacted accordingly. This still happens, of course; I understand it a bit better but essentially all that has changed is that I go my own way. I no longer feel lost behind that screen—which is not to imply that my frustration has disappeared.

The fact remains, however, that once labeled, there are powerful cultural forces at play. The label of disease does carry with it expectations of behavior. There is a sick role, so to speak.

There is a very low tolerance in this culture for ambiguity. We prefer situations to be defined, statuses to be clear. We want immediate answers and clear-cut resolutions. Our attention span is short—on both a national and a personal level. Once we think we have an answer, we would like to forget the question. We stereotype and classify because it is easier, because we do have difficulty with uncertainty, and because in many ways it is easier to deal with an idea of a person than with that individual. If I can classify you and reify you, then I don't have to *see* you, much less deal with your ever-changing and messy reality. There is, correspondingly, very little tolerance of those who float in and out of a role or a status. People do want certainty and, in search of that, attempt to pigeonhole each other. Once one is placed in that pigeonhole, people generally tend to want one to stay there. It can be difficult to resist that pressure.

On a day-to-day level, and even with those I am closest to, I find that the inherent instability of this disease and its ever-changing effects on me can enormously complicate life and relationships. A very small example of this comes from my tendency to walk into walls and lose my balance. There are many times, though, when my balance is fine. On those days, when I might stand on a chair and change a light bulb, I dislike intensely the fact that Nick watches me so closely in the fear that I might fall and that he worries. He, who knows me so well, has great difficulty with the uncertain effects of this disease on me. It would be much easier, in some ways, if I am to be sick that I be truly and unchangingly sick. And I do not want to be watched. Yet I have fallen many times in the last few years and I have always been glad when someone has picked me up. Nick assumes that I might fall and, as a result, is very protective and watchful. I assume I won't and want to be left alone. Yet I want someone ready to pick me up if I do fall. All very unreasonable.

Of course, this is all further complicated by my own understandings of who and what I am. I do not wish to be treated as though I am sick. However, I find that I would like people to quietly notice and make allowances on those days when normal functioning is very difficult. I resent equally those who make an enormous fuss over me and those who ignore my difficulty. I so clearly want it both ways and yet I am very aware of how unreasonable an expectation that is.

All of the above—roles, labeling, and their consequences—result from and are complicated by the assumptions and broad cultural values I identified. Underlying most of the conflicts I feel is the issue of strength and weakness, which I have come to see as the central dilemma posed for me by MS. This dilemma is shaped both by prevailing cultural values and my internalization of and response to those values. Going back to language, I am told that "handicapped" is an undesirable term because it connotes helplessness. Now, helplessness is an extreme state and I do not come close to approaching that. Yet my disease does impede my ability to function. Why then, the need to deny that? What is wrong with acknowledging weakness if it is real? And I do see in myself both that tendency and the ways in which it unnecessarily complicates my life.

I am sitting here at my word processor and my legs are feeling at one and the same time like lead and like cotton wool. I feel as though I shall never be able to move them again. (They do, however, move when I summon the energy—they have not yet ceased to be responsive.) Nick has taken my list and gone to the supermarket. He enjoys shopping; I do not. It would be difficult, today, for me to do that chore. He has, so far as I can tell, done it gladly. Yet I have trouble accepting his gift and as far as I know, it is my difficulty, not at all a problem for him. This is a minor but good example of one of the things I have had most trouble with in adjusting to the impact of MS. It interests me because I think if I fully understand exactly what is involved in a situation of this kind, I may be able to understand more clearly those situations which are not so minor.

I have great difficulty asking for help; I have difficulty (though to a lesser degree) accepting it. I don't want to be seen as a whiner; I certainly never want to use my weakness (however legitimate and real) as a manipulative tool. I don't want to be seen as weak even when I am weak. I think all of this flows out of my perception of how people in general interpret weakness. It also reflects my own acceptance on some level of the extremely negative cultural bias against weakness. A nonscientific survey of acquaintances showed that strength connotes good, active, competence, independence, hardness, and male. Weakness connotes passivity, illness, softness, bad, inadequate, and female. In this context I think it is clear that the stereotypes of women and of disability are reinforcing.

The strength/weakness dilemma has so many elements and is so complex and confusing that I have had great difficulty thinking it through. This is magnified by the reality that, for me, this is a continuing and daily conflict. It may seem to be clear and resolved and then I turn around and there it is again, usually in a new form. At its most basic, it is a question of maintaining integrity in the face of one's awareness that physical weakness is equated with, or at least inextricably entwined with, moral weakness. This dilemma seems a perfect example of acceptance as process; a continued living of acceptance and in that living, continued discovery.

Looking at my experience before and after my diagnosis, I assumed, as I have said, that much would be illuminated and clarified by that event. And there was some new clarity. But there were also new layers of cloud. Afterward, to be sure, my experience—redefined—was in a sense legitimated. My actions and perceptions were retroactively affirmed, my history given a different cast. There were, too, immediate benefits. My "weakness" was legitimated, but benefits always have their cost and I remain loath to claim them.

It became very clear—once an explanation of my history was available—exactly how loaded weakness is in this culture. Before my diagnosis it had not been enough for me to be who I was. There had been no acceptance of the reality that I was weak and sick. It had to be labeled and, hence, legitimized to be acceptable—culturally legitimated. In this culture, that demanded, in part, rational explanation. Because for years there was no rational explanation for my weakness, it was in a very real way unacceptable. Once there was a disease label attached to me, the external framework changed. Others' perceptions of me changed radically and, in their eyes, I was suddenly different. At first it seemed as though this was very straightforward. There were objective and legitimate explanations for my weakness. As the years passed, however, I became very aware of the limits to that clarity.

How naïve of me it was to think that a label would resolve everything. It merely moved everything to a new level, beyond me in some ways and in others, back to me. After receiving a diagnosis, the conflict between strength and weakness became more my conflict. Before then, I had been forcibly shaped by it, now it is more mine. But the structure of the conflict is clearer. Sickness itself is viewed, in a fairly covert way, as weakness—it has a moral cast. Weakness, however legitimate, is not legitimate.

I know, too, that it is precisely because of my history that even such "legitimated" weakness is difficult for me to deal with. I learned during all those years to expect that phrase, "It's all in your head." There is a level at which I am still wary of hearing that and tend to be defensive even when I need not be. And, as with the uncertainty, the power of the diagnosis as event to illuminate the issue of weakness has been shown with time to be limited. As on both sides of the diagnosis there was uncertainty, so on both sides there remains the issue of weakness. I view it differently; the prism did change. But here, too, while everything changed, everything remained the same.

The roots of this conflict are perhaps in the end not so very important. (For a brilliant discussion of the social construction of disease, see Susan Sontag's *Illness as Metaphor*.) Their significance to me reflects my full participation in the culturally constructed notion that there needs to be and that there is rationality in explanation. I have been intrigued by a notion which, as so many of these ideas do, strikes one as fresh and new but which, of course, is perfectly obvious once it has been pointed out. This notion is that there is a "fundamental incompatibility between the rationale for many customary ideas and rules, and our culturally constructed notion of rationality as a universal power of the mind unaffected by cultural variation."[2] I think this is very relevant here. Many of the values and, indeed, responses that I have been talking about are, perhaps, not either

2. Richard Handler, "Of Cannibals and Custom: Montaigne's Cultural Relativism, *Anthropology Today* (October 1986): 12–13.

rooted in or reducible to reason. And yet I find myself searching for those rational explanations or reasons; it is almost as if I believe that in reasonable explanation there is power.

One result of that continuing search is the knowledge that explanation, even when available, does fail. There is some comfort to be found in explanation but not, in the end, much power. Seeing the conflicts I feel and to some degree understanding their roots makes clear that while explanation does help, it clearly has its limits. Why is it so hard to acknowledge weakness? Once one sees why that is, shouldn't it then be easy to say OK, and move away from that? It doesn't seem to work that way. Understanding does not lead inevitably to resolution.

The central reality is that the constellation found in the concepts of strength and weakness presents me with, or creates for me, a daily and constant battle. Showing weakness, acknowledging it, is very difficult for me. My slowly emerging understanding of why that is does not always seem to change that reality. Again, this is in some measure because of my history; that is not something that fades easily. Beyond that and, of course, inextricably mixed with my own psychological makeup, are the cultural strands and, on an immediate level, the quality and content of interpersonal relationships.

As I have said before (but then it cannot be said too often), one of the difficulties with MS is that it can be generally invisible and there is no end to it; its legitimacy can therefore be doubtful. My statement of how I am feeling on a given day is not generally supported by anything visible. I have sometimes found myself longing for a broken leg. (And then thought, how completely neurotic.) But then I would have a very visible ailment, one with a discrete beginning and ending. People would respect that. I could legitimately go to bed for a week and rest. The fatigue associated with MS is almost invisible; there will always be those who question its reality and I find that very difficult.

An August weekend with close friends had been planned for months. I had committed myself to this visit and had a nonrefundable airplane ticket. The summer was long and hot and I had a progressively difficult time functioning. As the weekend approached, I was weaker than ever. I did not go on that trip; I lacked the strength. I wasn't sure that my friends understood. I was afraid that they thought I merely chose not to make that trip for other reasons. But because I know I tend to be defensive, having learned that many people do not see the effects of MS on me as constituting a valid excuse for anything, I was left uncertain. This is another example of how limited, in practice, the diagnosis turned out to be. The clarity I welcomed has its limits. And it becomes very circular—your reactions, my reactions to those, my *expectation* of your reactions—all of which tends to obscure what you are really thinking.

This is a self-propelled world in which things get done. Those who are well work and do all the other ordinary tasks of life whether or not they want to. If someone is sick, then they are given an exemption and there is no resentment. But if one is on the border, neither actively sick nor well, that is culturally problematic. The leaves do have to be raked (or so some people believe). One part of this dynamic that troubles me is its inherent potential for manipulation. It is very real; I am the only one who really knows how I feel on a given day, and it is not generally reflected in my appearance. I have, on occasion, used the excuse of MS to get out of things. I try very hard to be aware of this potential and to be manipulative only if I am conscious of it, but I think even that level of dishonesty creates problems. There is a point at which being conscious of the potential for manipulation and attempting to avoid it strikes me as in and of itself manipulative. A conundrum for which I have no answer.

At those times when I have been forced to use a cane to walk any distance, I have become aware that it acts as a labeler of sorts. It provides a level of explanation, as it were, that gives a sort of standing. If I stumble or fall using a cane, people do not react as though I am intoxicated. On the other hand, I am reluctant to use a cane even when I need one because I do not like being labeled or slotted. Legitimacy, yes, but one is then set apart and is face to face with common expectations of disease and disability. Costs and benefits—and another example of how much I want to have it both ways. Claiming the benefits requires clarity about the dynamics involved.

I think a part of the strength/weakness dilemma for me is directly related to this. It is exactly because the legitimacy of my weakness is in question that many times I have difficulty acknowledging it to others. Beyond that, I know that people have great difficulty with ambiguity. Once categorized, there is a whole set of common expectations of behavior that comes into play. These expectations differ as to disease and disability, as I said before. Disease is seen as having two outcomes—recovery or death. Disability is seen as being relatively stable and changing only for the worse. When one day I need a cane to walk with any ease and on the next I walk fairly normally, expectations are confounded. There is no slot into which I fit and that presents difficulties for me and for others. My status is not fixed. MS is a disease but it does not fit easily into folk categories of disease; it has disabled me but that disability is ever-changing and, moreover, is not always reflected in my appearance.

I have an extraordinarily difficult time calling my office to say I am sick. There are three related parts to this difficulty. The first is how to know myself whether on a given day I should rest or try to struggle through. The second is that I worry that I will not have enough sick leave when I need it. At those times when it is most difficult for me to function, I am most reluctant to use sick leave because I am afraid I will need it more next week or next month. The weaker I am, the more I wonder if I will be even weaker later on. The third reason for my reluctance is a lingering feeling that I will be suspected of malingering. I am most apt to call in sick on Fridays, which is logical enough because during a period of reintensification each succeeding day takes its toll. But everyone (and with reason) is suspicious of a worker taking sick leave on a Friday. The result of all this is that I feel defensive even when there is not only no real reason for it but when the people around me are very supportive and give me no reason to think they distrust me. Once again, I create the difficulty for myself.

Because strength and weakness are so loaded in this culture and so bound up with our notions of maleness and femaleness, individuality and independence, when one is neither physically strong nor weak but in a constant state of flux, there are continuing social consequences. I have sometimes thought that if only things would stay the same, I could more easily adjust. But, of course, that is not the case. It is only as I have begun to understand how strong are the templates we carry in our minds—and they are all slightly different—of what disease and disability mean and their implications and how difficult it is to go beyond them that I can begin to accept those implications. It is not particularly easy for me to have to struggle to walk one day and the next walk fairly easily. I can't categorize myself. How much harder it is for those around me.

There is another aspect to the conflicts I feel surrounding the issue of strength and weakness that seems to be common among those I have talked to about this issue. It is a very intense feeling that if one gives in to weakness, one will become weaker. I find that on those days when I am weakest, my instinctive response seems to be to try to do more. That response, I believe, arises out of the fear of dependence, and that fear has a lot to do with the strong negative connotations of dependence in this culture.

Dependence is not something we in this culture easily or openly acknowledge. We prefer to ignore or mask the fact that we are all dependent in many unavoidable and, indeed, good ways. Independence is a highly desired and valued goal; it is closely related to the centrality of the individual and all that flows therefrom. We cherish independence and strength and they are closely entwined—strength is viewed as leading to or permitting independence. Conversely, weakness leads to dependence and both are seen as highly undesirable states. Notwithstanding that true mutuality, involving both independence and dependence, is a *sine qua non* of life and of all interpersonal relationships, our mythology glorifies individual independence.

There is, too, a crucial distinction between physical and nonphysical dependence. On an individual level, it seems that when I was not dependent, I could be dependent or that when I was strong, weakness was, in a sense, permissible. The difference seems to lie in the fact of one's real and physical dependence; the illusion, for that is what it is, of choice is lost. One is unable to retain the belief that if only one chose, one could be independent. And it is exactly because I am dependent in new ways and, more crucially, potentially dependent, that I fight against it. When dependence was not so real, I could more easily achieve true mutuality in relationships—giving and taking and needs were more balanced. Now there is an area in which I continue to be dependent and it skews the balance.

I am reminded of the *berdache* of certain North American Indian groups. The *berdache* were men who voluntarily took on the role and status of women and who were so regarded by their community. They were reputed to be excellent wives. They were said to perform women's tasks better than the women did because they were still men and were expected to excel in all things. They could be good women because they were not women. I could deal with dependence when I was not (in such a clear-cut way) dependent; now that I am, and independence is not an option, I am not very good at it at all.

Quite clearly at play here are power and control and fear. On a grand scale, I have no illusions of my ability to control much of anything, nor do I have any real desire to do so. On a lower-level daily scale, I do want to be in control. Asking for help inevitably involves a loss of control. It also requires openness and a subjection to another's construction of reality. I resist that. My clarity about what is involved and its necessity does not altogether ease that resistance. I want to control my living environment and I do not want to give over to another power over my daily life. My greatest fear is of becoming so disabled that I lose the ability to control my daily life.

One day while I was sitting in my yard with a friend, my kitten ran up a tree. As kittens are wont to do, she quickly decided that going up was one thing, coming down altogether different. My friend said, "Oh leave her, she'll come down eventually." I couldn't convince him to rescue her and so I climbed up the tree. And then discovered that I could not get back down. My legs were shaking uncontrollably and I had lost all sense of their position. My friend then had to rescue me and the cat— after he stopped laughing. And it was a very funny moment. I should have known better than to climb that tree. I do not like to admit that there are things I cannot do but more than that, I dislike relinquishing control even on that level. My cat, my tree, and if I lacked the ability to rescue her, she would not be rescued. The resolution of that situation would have been out of my hands if I admitted, as I should have done, my inability to rescue her. Oh yes, a very minor example, but important to me. I do not want to lose the ability to decide and control those small things. This represents a continuing struggle for me. Awareness of what is involved does not seem to resolve it. The best I can do so far is to try to be aware and to keep the outline of the conflict in my mind.

I also, of course, fear the effects of weakness and physical dependency on relationships. There is the danger that if I show you who I really am, you will reject me, and if I ask something of you, you will turn away. I think most of us are prone to believe this at one time or another—unconditional love and acceptance are truly rare. I like to think that I have gone beyond that and in effect, say to people, this is who I am and what you do with that is fine. Nevertheless, when I think of the possibilities inherent in this disease, those fears do recur. The other aspect, and the much more tangible one, is that regardless of the level of trust, love, and acceptance in any relationship, there is inevitably going to be at least occasional anger and resentment when one person is continually physically needy. For me, it is absolutely essential to have that reality acknowledged and brought out in the open and that requires new levels of trust and acceptance.

For me it sometimes seems as though the hardest thing I have to do is to acknowledge my weakness; does one have to be strong to be weak? Is that a reflection of my personal psychological makeup? Indubitably; however, I do think that it has much more to do with the tone and values of this culture. If my weakness is objective and legitimate, why must it be masked with strength? Would it be more culturally acceptable for me to be weak if I were in fact strong? Or, put another way, if I deny my weakness and my need for help, do I then become a "better" weak person?

This may have something to do with being a woman. I wonder whether a man, generally perceived as stronger and more independent purely because of his sex, would have an easier time coming to terms with dependence. As with the *berdache*, because he is not dependent, he could be dependent. Because he is a man, he is strong; asking for help, therefore, is not a reflection of weakness. Women who continue to be, at least covertly, perceived as passive and dependent perhaps find it more difficult to acknowledge dependence. It must also be remembered that women, traditionally dependent and passive (at least theoretically), exercised great if covert power through manipulating that role. I am very wary of finding myself in that position. An argument can be made that acknowledging dependence is harder for men because of the cultural prohibitions against showing weakness and because they tend to have less explicit experience with it. Nevertheless, I do think there is a very real sense in which the converse is true.

At the root of all of this remains the cultural framework in which illness, disability, and dependence are equated with moral weakness and failure. It was one thing entirely to identify that framework and another to begin to come to terms with my own responses to it. My fear of being seen as weak and dependent in large part arises out of my view of the culture's judgment of those conditions. I do not wish to be judged a moral failure. Notwithstanding that I question those values, I still find that judgment hard to bear. It is precisely because weakness is so adversely viewed that I sometimes feel an almost irresistible need to mask it. From my perspective, it has seemed as though it does require strength to acknowledge weakness, to ask for help. And yet asking for help when it is necessary is something I must be able to do. I would like there to be more congruence between what living with multiple sclerosis requires of me on a daily basis and the way in which I am judged by society. At root, the strength to be weak involves resisting others' interpretation of my experience and finally, because that resistance is not very useful, letting it go and accepting the conflict as given.

I feel very strongly that in many ways the culture (that grand abstraction) would have me believe that my disease reflects the imperfection of my nature and indicates a lack of control where there should be control. Beyond that, it would have me believe in a better tomorrow; never stop trying to "do something about it;" and above all value and fight for my independence. The very curious thing is that I never did believe those things or subscribe to those values and, as time passes, I feel more and more at odds with the general thrust of this culture. Why then, am I so damned concerned with these things now?

When you are weak and dependent in many ways and live in a society which glorifies strength and independence, there is inevitably a conflict. I think a natural response is to deny one's weakness. I want to be accepted as I am and yet, when I acknowledge weakness or ask for help, I immediately am covered over, as it were, by the blanket of others' conscious and unconscious understandings of what that means. Of course, this statement is both greatly oversimplified and disregards much of what occurs on an individual level. But I think in a very general way it explains some of what lies behind or even requires denial. The language and the dynamics of denial—fighting against, not giving in, overcoming—and its other side—giving in—reflect not only the individual experience but a social experience, a social reality.

A young man in his twenties, whose leg had been amputated at a much earlier age, was found at a Neanderthal burial site at Shanidar in Iraq.[3] To survive, this man must have been cared for by his community. Moreover, the decision to amputate (to save his life?) must have been accompanied by a community decision to provide such care. In one of the earliest human communities we know of, people were caring for a man who had to have been, given what we know of that culture, totally dependent on them. We know of no animals who care for each other in such ways. It raises fascinating questions. Did these people commonly care for each other in this way, or did this individual possess knowledge that was critical to the community's survival? I wonder how much of what I feel, he felt. Did he feel the **conflicts that I feel, or perhaps, different ones? And I wonder, too, about his place in that community. What was his social** reality?

3. Eric Trinkhaus, *The Shanidar Neanderthals* (New York: Academic Press, 1983).

MS, or any chronic disease, presents an obstacle. It is a real and objective obstacle. It cannot be overcome; it must be accepted. Yet I find that my own acceptance is not enough. I must also accept the cultural consequences of that acceptance.

So in the end, there seem to be two separate elements bound up in my struggle with weakness and dependence. And I am not at all sure which is stronger. There is the fear of dependence and there is the fear of being seen as dependent. Although I would prefer to think of myself as one who is not concerned with what "people" will think, it is quite obvious that my difficulty stems in large measure from exactly that. I begin to believe that this is another, perhaps less obvious, reflection of that uncertainty I tried to describe earlier. Why is it that I am now more concerned with the opinions of others? It is a direct outgrowth of my uncertainty, a reflection of new vulnerability and fear of dependence. It is because of all that that I seem now to require more affirmation.

The convergence of these fears may have much to do with that illusion we have of choice and control and the ways in which it operates. When it was theoretically possible for me, if I so chose, to fully participate in this society, it was quite easy for me to reject it. Now that I am an outsider, it is harder for me to be an outsider. When it was possible for me to be congruent with my culture and I chose not to do so, that was one thing; now that it is impossible, I suddenly find it problematic. Or is that just a reflection of the general perversity of human nature? I always did feel an outsider in many ways and for many reasons and never was troubled by that. I had no desire to be an insider, or to belong to something whose central ethos and values I questioned. I still do question those values; they are not my values, yet I find that in some ways I almost wish they were.

Perhaps it all returns to the question of denial. It may be at the very root of denial. That because there is conflict between the culture and what is required of me on a daily basis, and because acknowledgment of that requires great clarity and discomfort, the simplest thing, the way to live in some psychological comfort and congruity with one's culture, is to deny the conflict, which means denying the full implications of disease, potential dependence, lack of control, and ultimately, of course, mortality. I can't do that, I don't even want to do that, but the conflicts are real and continuing. Understanding their causes and roots does help, but issues like dependence or strength and weakness will continue to be issues for me, I imagine. The terms of the struggle do and will continue to change. My understanding and my acceptance may increase. In this regard, however, it begins to seem that acceptance is acceptance of the conflict as a continuing part of my life.

# Beyond Acceptance

The acceptance process is much more complex than I thought. It is not just a question of me and my responses and acceptance or nonacceptance of having MS. There is not only me alone adjusting to my new reality and all that encompasses. It is not merely that I can no longer rely on my legs not to buckle and all the psychological consequences of that. Suddenly, I am face to face with the expectations, classifications, categorizations, and stereotypical reactions of others. There is a whole world to adjust to, and that world makes acceptance and adjustment more complicated than if I lived in isolation.

It is, in many ways, the various social aspects of the process which are most problematic. An important part of that world is the relationship with one's physician. That relationship is an important one in and of itself for anyone with a chronic illness. It is also in many ways a perfect example of the whole world of relationships. Since my diagnosis, I have begun to think that the physician-patient relationship is open to misunderstanding in some measure because of the values and assumptions I have been talking about. We tend to bring that framework with us—it would be strange if we did not—into our relations with doctors and we also overlay those relations with a set of mostly unspoken and even unrealized expectations.

I have often wondered why doctors play down the impact of being told that one has a disease such as multiple sclerosis. I think the answer is partly found in the ramifications of the meaning of time. Time and perceptions of time (its presence and passage) are central in both the experience of disease and in responses to it. It is central to others' perceptions and responses; it is central to my own. Time, of course, is not the right word at all. I don't mean time in the sense of its divisions or as implying passage. Time (or is it our experience of time) is always in motion, not necessarily toward or from but in rearrangement of the molecules—Brownian motion—molecules randomly colliding and moving in response to those collisions.

We tend to fix people in time and then respond to our picture of them. We disregard, often because we do not know, how they may have changed from that fixed picture and how they may have experienced the time that has passed. I think of speaking on the telephone to a dearly loved friend after a few days; I know where I have been in those days, how the atoms of reality have rearranged themselves. But not only do I not know where he has been, what he has done, how he has changed, I must actively remember that I do know none of that. For if I fail to know that, I lose the capacity to hear him or be with him where he is at that moment.

Time is, perhaps, one aspect of the doctor-patient relationship which, being at least tacitly, if not actively, misunderstood, contributes to the potential difficulties in that relation. My neurologist is a very sensitive and compassionate man. He listens very carefully, a rare quality. But his knowledge of me is necessarily limited. (Because that knowledge is, in large part, based on my presentation, I am responsible for it.) His experience of me is based on discrete episodes, fixed in time, while who I am at that moment is only one part of a continuum.

It may be just because doctors do see only moments, isolated from life, from relationships, that they tend to understate the importance of the disease for the patient. "So you can't walk very well," and seen purely objectively, I would not disagree. But for me there is nothing objective nor isolated about that fact.

Akin to this is something that I feel very strongly every time I see my neurologist. I have a benign form of this disease. He deals every day with acutely and grievously ill people. In his world, I am clearly one of the lucky ones. Seen through his eyes,

I am quite well. In my world—and especially compared to the way I used to be—I am not OK at all. I try to remember that. It is, in part, a question of perspectives. For me, it is of major importance that many days I must struggle to walk. In his world, I walk very well. But it is also a matter exactly of the existence of those separate worlds. For me, it is I who am central; we are all central in our own worlds and, I think, often forget that we are central nowhere else. It is important to remember those different worlds.

I think of a day when I was walking along and suddenly felt something very strange or, rather, I felt nothing at all and wondered if my shoe had broken. Well, my shoe was fine. My ankle had collapsed and there was no sensation attached to that event. There was suddenly no support there. I reported this to my doctor and he said, "Oh yes, that was an ankle collapse." For him, it was another transient symptom; for me, it was much more. I wanted to say to him, "Hey, wait. This is important to me." I didn't because this man is the only doctor in my experience who almost never downplays the importance of what is happening. And for once, I did remember the essential difference in our perspectives.

Nevertheless, there is something very unsettling about that kind of thing. A fundamental disturbance of body image. I think of reports I have heard from those who have been through earthquakes. After the earth, the very ground—that immutable and permanent element—has moved, it is hard to trust in the certainty of anything. Comparing an ankle collapse to an earthquake is perhaps farfetched but I think the ensuing feelings are related. I can no longer trust that my ankle will not collapse; I can't assume anything about it. For me, and I am not sure why this particular symptom did affect me so strongly (perhaps it was the absence of all feeling, the ankle lay there on the floor and it was only vision that told me so), it was quite like an earthquake.

Disturbance of body image is very shattering. It disturbs the very experience and root of self. I think one has no real awareness of the centrality to self of that body image or, indeed, no awareness that one holds that image, until it is disturbed. I often think with awe of the many years in which I was so completely unaware of the fact that my legs worked. One takes so much for granted.

As I looked at that ankle, lying sideways on the floor, it felt completely unconnected to me. Yet, of course, it remained a part of me. Communication was disturbed. Another example of this and, in its way, even more compelling has to do with movement. There have been times walking when suddenly I have stopped, not as a result of intention but because my left leg has ceased to move, to take the next step. And then one has to think about it, to actively think, to will, movement. Unthought, unconscious movement has ceased.

When my left side is numb or in whatever fashion "not right," I always have my right side as a reference point. I have wondered what it would be like if they were both the same. Sometimes I think it is only or partly because my right side is there, is normal, that I am aware of the left-side deficits.

These events can be medically simple and objectively (if that is even a category here) straightforward and of a minor nature. Yet they do shake the ground, as it were, for an individual. Such sensations, or the lack thereof, are clearly connected to that generalized uncertainty I spoke of before. The psychological consequences of the physical events are so much more important than the events in and of themselves.

It is difficult to convey their impact. Perhaps unless one has experienced something of this kind, one really cannot comprehend its nature. I surely never thought before of how right my body felt, or was grateful that my legs obeyed commands I never was aware of giving. As may be true in the aftermath of an earthquake, one becomes aware through loss, or change, of that which one had not consciously known as such before. I certainly don't appreciate the stability of the ground beneath my feet as I walk down the street.

Perhaps when something of this nature happens to us and so overshadows everything else, our self-absorption becomes so great (I have felt sometimes as though I must listen to, and could hear, the internal workings of my body) that we tend not to want to hear how commonplace it really is. And that there is nothing anyone could say that would convince us we were being taken seriously enough.

Another factor affecting the patient-doctor relationship may result from the explosion in medical research and technology. We have learned to expect that something will be done, that action can be taken, results assured. So much is possible now that was unthought of just a few years ago. MS presents a case where not much can be done or given. Playing it down may be a response to this fact. I think most doctors would like to be able to do something for their patients; in addition, I think most patients expect that something will be done. There is a tendency to see doctors as very powerful. A disease such as MS with an uncertain course, an uncertain prognosis, no cure, and only palliative treatment available, confounds that relationship. I think the common assumption that all problems have a solution, that anything is possible, is particulary active and powerful in this context. Here, where the problem has no solution and everything is not possible, there may well be conflict. Doctors may have trouble acknowledging their impotence and their patients may be unable to admit to themselves that there is no affirmative action available.

I am aware that despite my best efforts these assumptions lurk in the background whenever I see my neurologist. I see him because I have reached the temporary end of my ability to cope. As he once pointed out, I never call him just to say hello, how are you. No patient does. And, if I am honest, I call him because I want something to be done. This is so even though I know perfectly well that nothing can be done. There is, at least, covertly, a request from me to him to do something; I would not be there otherwise. What he gives me is information and reassurance. That is extremely important, and I don't discount its value for a minute. What is important, though, is the way in which I continue, in the face of my own clear understanding, to (at least on some level) expect some action. Whenever there is a request, however hidden, there is equally an expectation of response. And I think it is because we are acculturated in action, in resolution, and in change that, despite our best efforts, we find it difficult, when necessary, to shrug off that response.

Notwithstanding my attempts to understand and be conscious of what motivates me and shapes my responses, all of this can be, at times, enormously frustrating. Another of my doctors believes that my disease is so benign that it should not be a factor in my life at all. I have often wished that he could spend a day, one of the bad days, in my body. When doctors deny the impact of disease, for whatever reasons, some of which may be quite valid in their eyes—for example, a desire to ease the impact and promote acceptance—adjustment becomes even more difficult. At least for me, it is much harder to come to terms with something if I am the only one who thinks it important. That response feeds the general uncertainty. One thinks, "Perhaps this really shouldn't matter, perhaps I am overreacting," and so forth. This itself can be a crucial element in denial.

The patient-doctor relationship is one example—and central to the chronically ill—of the whole world of relationships. Life with chronic disease exists on a continuum. One has to remember that the quality and content of that continuum cannot be easily conveyed to others. We always see of others only discrete episodes.

The centrality of denial in so many responses to disease can be explained by the interaction of (at least short-term) individual psychological needs and the impact of culture. Both reinforce the other and, indeed, give each other more power. Of course, one might well argue that culture reflects—is derived from—individual needs and I think that is true. The converse, that individual psychology reflects culture, is probably true, too, but to a lesser degree. Words such as culture represent abstractions which should not be given spurious reality. I do not mean to imply that such concepts are active and moving forces or have reality in and of themselves. Nevertheless, I do think there is an important interactive process at work here which cannot be ignored.

It is commonly held that denial is an inevitable and necessary stage in the acceptance process. I have not found that to be the case. Shock and disbelief, yes, but those emotions are not to be equated with denial. I have wondered if perhaps hope and denial are so closely entwined that each is to be found only in the presence of the other. And that because I did not have (what I would deem false) hope, neither was I impelled to denial. Equally, because I felt no drive to deny the reality of what was happening to me, I did not seek refuge in hope.

I don't know what individual characteristics promote or even require denial. I do know that even though I skipped that stage, I have felt, and continue to feel, the force of the imperative to deny. It also seems as though the denial of others is an obstacle I continually run up against. These concepts seem, for many, to carry within them their own truth and power. I have been intrigued by those who say, "You are denying the fact of this disease." When I say, "No, I don't think so," I am told that my statement that I am not engaging in denial proves that I am. There seems to be a commonly held appreciation of the reality, necessity, and universality of both hope and denial. It is here, I think, that an explanation is to be found for the misperception of acceptance as event. Moreover, the belief that acceptance will preclude conflict and negative feelings is bound to affect the individual. For as one continues (and one will) to experience conflict, one may well feel a need to deny that experience.

I think, too, that we are sidetracked by semantics. I feel very strongly (as is probably more than clear) that the emphasis on hope and denial and their centrality in most discussions of illness and death grievously impairs acceptance. But many of those I have discussed this with have taken violent issue with me. Hope is a very loaded word. Questioning the use of hope seems almost as bad as attacking motherhood. It is not entirely clear to me exactly what many people mean when using that word. It seems sometimes to be shorthand for an optimistic and positive outlook on life; it obviously has strong religious overtones; it holds within it the notion of change.

The fact that hope, as generally used, precludes acceptance is disregarded. I am a fairly cheerful and, at root, very happy person, happy especially in the little things. I see great joy in life itself. And yet I find repeatedly that if I express a lack of hope, or perhaps, more accurately, indicate that hope is not a centerpiece of my world view, I am assumed to be in despair. There seems to be an equation of clear and straightforward acceptance with pessimism, even depression. It is intriguing that while both "despairing" and "despondent" are listed synonyms for "hopeless," the primary definition is "giving no grounds for hope." There is a common understanding (is it reflective of or structured by language?) at work here which is difficult to get around. Does the absence of hope necessarily create a hole to be filled with despair? Clearly I don't think so. Nevertheless, it has become clear to me that viewing acceptance as a continuing and ever-evolving process with no clear end and certainly no resolution of conflict is often equated with despair.

In this vein, it has been pointed out to me that hope, rather than being an avoidance technique or a tool of denial, is a coping mechanism. Undoubtedly, that is true. It seems to me, however, that if it is a coping mechanism, my point is made. It is exactly because hope is used as a way around reality, a refuge, a way of dealing with that which we would prefer not to deal with at all, that it gets in our way.

The following prescription seems a fair statement of and reflection of the ways in which both hope and denial are commonly used. While it was written in the context of life-threatening disease, I think it applies equally here:

> Hope is necessary . . . for sustaining a sense of oneself as a person with a future; without that expectation, the experience would be one of despair only. Denial—of death and of the immediate limits imposed by the disease—is necessary to the idea of oneself as someone who exists apart from the condition of illness, whose true self continues distinct throughout and emerges intact at the end.[1]

I find the implications of this statement for acceptance to be appalling. Specifically, the notion that denial is necessary is destructive. I do not exist apart from my disease; wherever the boundaries of self and body are to be found, the only way I can live is with full acceptance that this disease is a permanent part of me. There can be no integration otherwise. I am intact, yes, and that is essential, but that intactness is of the whole and the

1. Martha Fay, *A Mortal Condition* (New York: Coward-McCann, 1983), p. 18.

whole includes the disease. And as for the future, there is a sense in which we all assume a future; no matter how accepting of our mortality we may be, we do tend to trust that there will be a tomorrow. My sense of personal integrity, of existence, is not at all dependent on hope. Tomorrow is unknown, uncertain and, other than in necessary and practical ways, in no way governs today. And I imagine that if I had knowledge of my certain and impending death, that would be even more true. If denial is necessary and reliance on hope essential, it all becomes a game.

Death is at the root of our conceptions and understanding of both hope and denial. Certainly, it is apparent to a casual observer of this culture that death is dealt with in the most obfuscatory fashion. I suppose that if death is a fact we prefer to obscure, then it follows that anything tending to remind us of our mortality will also be obscured. MS, or any disease, is necessarily and foremost a reminder of our mortal nature even though it may not be immediately life-threatening.

Death is the ultimate reminder of our lack of control. That fact, however, and its commonness remains something which we prefer to ignore. It might be argued that the very supremacy and centrality of the belief that man can control nature, can change outcomes, is only a reflection of our, however covert, acceptance of our mortality. It is because we do know that we will die that we are so preoccupied by death and try so hard to overcome it through activity. Control is so important exactly because deep down we do know we have no control.

For me, masking that fact—that we are mortal, that we have finite lives—makes living rather futile, removes what point there is to be found. Remove the sacred canopy—whatever it is created out of, hope, religion—and there is reality and, hence, life. To ignore death takes away a large part of life's joy. It is within the "immediate limits imposed"—the constraints and the real context of my life seen through clear eyes—that there is room for a full life and for happiness.

I have been concerned with the process of adjustment to the knowledge that one has, and will continue to have, a chronic disease. Before there can be adjustment, however, there must be acceptance of the very real conflicts inherent in and the limits imposed by MS. If it is, indeed, necessary to deny the very real limits and conflicts inherent in disease, there will be no acceptance. Adjustment is difficult enough; to try to adjust to something which one has successfully hidden from one's self is a continuing exercise in futility. There are plenty of people around who will support that exercise. Acceptance is in many ways and by many people equated with despair.

Beyond self and immediate others is always the world I live in and with, and I do find living in that world to be problematic. I have no desire or need to deny on a personal level; in fact, I have a very strong desire and need to be absolutely clear and honest about the consequences, real and potential, of MS for me. But I do feel rather strongly the pull to denial on a cultural level. I can easily see, too, how these two strands might become inextricably mixed. And when they do, clarity becomes even harder to find and retain.

I do resist being categorized by others. I dislike being put in the sick/disabled category and role. Physical weakness is difficult to accept. Weakness is undesirable; if it is seen as legitimate, it is better, but the visible results of MS, my condition, are often not seen that way. And because weakness and dependence are so negatively viewed, one has, or I have at least at times, a strong impulse to do whatever is necessary to avoid being seen and treated in that negative way. So, on that level, perhaps I do engage in denial. And it is obvious that that need and that response can lead back to individual denial. As I have become more aware of that dynamic, I have certainly appreciated in a new way the power of the external world to inform experience.

Trying to find a new job pointed out to me—if I had needed to have it pointed out, and by then I really did not—another way that denial is almost forced on the individual. I had had the notion that I had an obligation to tell a potential employer about my MS, that while I was generally well and quite able to perform my job, there were those bad days, days when walking was difficult and so forth. I felt, too, that I wanted my employer to know about the MS because if my condition deteriorated, I did not want that to come as a surprise. I was applying for jobs in which presumably the quality of my brain, not my body, was at issue. In none of the situations in which I was open about my MS was I offered a job. Of course, there is no way of knowing whether MS was the reason but I am fairly sure that it was. I stopped being honest about MS and I got a job. A friend who is very reticent about his MS cites employment as the primary reason and I have no reason to think he is wrong.

I think it becomes very difficult to be open and honest with one's self if one is, or feels compelled to be, secretive and dishonest with others. Honesty is not, after all, a two-sided thing. It either exists or it does not. A social imperative to denial inevitably will affect one on all levels, and it operates in many ways, through language, in relationships, through me. Acceptance, as commonly understood, is a perfect example.

It is difficult to maintain integrity in the face of these pressures. But it is impossible unless there is clarity about exactly what is at play. I think there is a way in which the society (and I do hesitate to throw around these abstractions) demands, perhaps through a tautological process, reaffirmation of its primary values. That which conflicts with the general thrust of society is, in a sense, brushed aside. It is important to hold to the centrality of my own reality, to remember the conflicts, and to remember also that neither my reality nor the social world will change. Life must be within that frame.

A partial explanation of this tautological process may be found in language itself. I think that language does structure experience. We tend to see things for which we have words and concepts; we place events within available categories. Beyond that, expectations create experience. Those expectations also arise out of language. Our expectations, however formed, can in large measure determine how we experience what happens to us. If we have a set of categories or visions within or through which we see the world, we will tend to place our experience within those categories, rather than seeing it as it is. An example is the way in which disease tends to be equated with sickness. As I have come to appreciate, disease not associated with sickness is anomalous. That categorization is not really very useful, yet it dominates and limits our understanding. Moreover, we use words to minimize and control uncertainty.

Thinking about language can become very circular and perhaps one never can see purely. How can one perceive reality other than through language? One intuitively senses language's inadequacy to describe or account for many things, but one is still limited by it. To give a small example, a friend pointed out to me that I seem to be creating an evolving category of good days and bad days to convey information in my closest relationships. If asked on a bad day, I have usually said that I am not very well. I have not said I am sick because being "sick" doesn't seem an apt description to me. But I have learned that "not being very well" doesn't seem to convey much to others. So I have relied more and more on the good-and-bad-day classification. This is one response to the inadequacy of existing categories. It is also a way of limiting expectations to daily realities, which I have tried to do although I doubt they can be done away with altogether. I do think that they can be very determinative of experience. I want the quality of my life to be as unfiltered by conscious or unconscious expectations as possible and to experience it as it is.

A dominant theme such as hope or denial does operate to shape our understanding. I must be aware of the ways in which I respond to the culture's treatment of disease and disability and my occasional desire to hide from that. Only then can I avoid disguising and distorting my own reality from myself. If I am aware of the ways in which my environment pulls me to and seduces me into thinking I have control over the facts of my life and denying my personal reality, I can better resist that pressure.

All of these factors are ongoing impediments to adjustment, perhaps even to acceptance, and they act in concert with those primary motivating values of this culture which do, and actively, conflict with my reality.

I must live in the present; this culture is strongly oriented to the future.

I must accept that I have no control over nature; this culture operates on the premise that nature is controllable.

I must accept that my independence and self-sufficiency are potentially in doubt and I must maintain my integrity in the face of that.

I must accept that, while action is the primary and almost

instinctive response in all situations, I must be with this disease.

A central requirement of both acceptance and adjustment is that one refashion one's conception of integrity, of personal wholeness. Before one can integrate the various impacts of the disease into a new vision of self, and go on from there, one must be fully aware of the entire set of consequences. You can't put something in its proper place until you know exactly what it is. It is only as I accept (and it does continue) the present and potential consequences of having MS, that I can then adjust to it. Without that acceptance, adjustment would be impossible; there would be nothing to adjust to, there would be only an unexamined, uncertain complex held away from myself. I think that the importance of this process is not only generally downplayed, but that much of my world tells me, in however obscure a fashion, don't do it. So, finally, acceptance requires conscious awareness of the action of that world. One must adjust to and accept the fact that acceptance and adjustment are not really seen as important or essential.

Acceptance also requires accepting that one will live at odds with the "onward and upward" thrust of this culture. Full individual acceptance requires a set of values that conflicts with prevailing values. I think that here is to be found a partial explanation of the prevalence of both hope and denial. We do want in some ways (comfort requires) to live in congruence with our culture. Yet integrity demands acknowledgment on an individual level of that which everything around us denies. The values of many people conflict with those that are dominant in society; mine did long before my diagnosis. The difference for me now lies in the acuteness of that conflict, as well as in the consequences of ignoring it. It is because alienation not only becomes so extreme but at the same time becomes intolerable in a new way because of one's new vulnerability that recognition of this conflict is essential. I doubt that resolution is possible.

The diagnosis, that event which even now seems such a central and clear demarcation of my experience, did not provide the resolution I thought was available. That moment of perfect clarity, while in many ways transforming my experience, ultimately failed both as explanation and as an agent of change.

What was central before my diagnosis, trying to live with integrity in a world shaped by others' interpretation of my experience, was central afterward. The definition and size of that world changed. The terms changed, the ground shifted, but the essential reality remained. And the scene at the airport in Luxor continues to be a very powerful metaphor for me of my experience on both sides of the diagnosis. The central issue is that of maintaining personal integrity and shaping one's own experience within the world, however defined.

And what, after all, is the hope of? While I would not use the word "waiting," for that holds its own implications, I do agree with T. S. Eliot that hope would be for the wrong thing. As I began to suspect on first reading the books about MS, it is always hope of change. It seems clearer and clearer to me that hope precludes living fully and completely today. It blurs reality; it takes the edge off; and finally, it makes acceptance almost beside the point. And acceptance of that which cannot be changed is essential. Only then can one adjust to what is and live fully as an integrated whole.

There was indeed a connection between the assumptions that bothered me so in what I read after my diagnosis and the fact that what I experienced was not addressed. For the values I have discussed do, if one holds them, obviate the need for real acceptance and even, to a degree, foreclose it. Beyond that, there is a reluctance which I appreciate, to say, "Wait a minute, this is my experience and I won't have it gainsaid." Coupled with that is a tendency to frame one's experience in terms that others both recognize and consider legitimate. Presumably one purpose (it is mine) of writing these books is to share one's experience, and there is concern that if that experience is contrary to common frames of reference, it will be misunderstood, if not disregarded. Intensifying that feeling is the vulnerability and uncertainty that causes me to question my own perceptions and understandings of this experience.

While I find that I have become increasingly impatient with and amused by self-absorption on all levels and try very hard to guard against it in myself, this book is in many ways an exercise in exactly that. I walk the streets and listen in on the floating scraps of conversation and am so often struck by how bound each of us is by our own small world—a private world unknowable to the observer but whose existence is palpably real. I feel sometimes as though we are all in crystal balls within which we live and through which we fail to see. These crystal balls, and the worlds they enclose, prevent us from entering fully into the world of another. Our individual worlds seem so important to us, so compelling, we fail to remember how small and limited they really are. And we do this on all levels, from the very personal to the most global. I had thought that viewing the earth from space—itself another entity floating, enclosed—would perhaps cure us of our sense of importance but that has not seemed to happen.

My world is not yours; nor yours mine. But if we both remember that neither world defines reality and that there need not be that opaque and enclosing wall, then perhaps we can begin truly to see and hear one another.

I do not want to fall into the trap of seeing reality only through the prism of MS. It has seemed important to understand the ways in which it is relevant and the ways in which the culture shapes my experience. It is all much clearer to me now. Receiving a diagnosis did illuminate and transform the past for me and coming back from Egypt did throw new light on my life with a chronic illness in this culture. The explanation I found for some of the conflicts I experience is very important. The conflicts do remain, however, and there is a very finite limit to the relevance or usefulness of that understanding. Clarity, even explanation, does not provide resolution.

The diagnosis, that watershed event, failed in the end in its promise of clarity and resolution. It was transforming; it did change everything. But equally, it changed nothing. Yes, I as an individual was affirmed and that was important. Acceptance on an individual level is crucial but does not provide closure.

I think I have, in the larger sense, accepted what MS means to me. The conflicts remain, however, and I rather think always will. It is possible to live with ease in the presence of those conflicts but only after accepting the full implications of their continuing existence. Living with chronic illness in this society will always require new adjustment. I doubt there will ever be any conclusion or closure to be found in this experience. The central and essential nature of acceptance—that it is a process and that it does not negate conflict—must be acknowledged. But it is important to state that in acknowledging conflict one can then, in a sense, go beyond it. These conflicts are not the central nor the most important fact about my life.

Having a disease of this nature is not separable from the rest of life. It is not something that can be segregated or held apart. All experience is viewed through that prism. It is not entirely a negative screen; I have found clarity (scattered and obscured though it may be) in observing myself and others through the overlay of this experience. But the prism is there and to ignore it is to deny myself the opportunity to live wholly and in integration.

The boundaries we create for ourselves, and the definitions, are ultimately very limiting. They do bind us and bound us. And just as I have great difficulty seeing the ultimate importance of divisions based on nationalism or other categories, so do I not wish to define myself in terms of MS nor take it too seriously.

Multiple sclerosis is only one part of me. The experience I have described is only one part of me. There is a whole world and a whole life beyond multiple sclerosis. To go beyond MS does require first seeing and accepting the continuing implications and consequences of a life framed by disease and understanding their roots.

It concerns me that to a degree the very process of acceptance—most particularly the describing of it—almost requires that it be given a stress that, in the end, is misleading, even false. There is life beyond MS. There is much joy and happiness in that life. With Virginia Woolf, I believe in the importance of the things one does not say. Beyond MS, there is always and foremost, "the question of things happening, normally, all the time."

Designed by Martha Farlow

Composed by G & S Typesetters, Inc., in Aster

Printed by R. R. Donnelley & Sons Company on 55-lb. Cream White Sebago
and bound in Holliston Roxite A with Rainbow Textured endsheets